Clinicians' Guide to
Oesophageal Diseases

Clinicians' Guide to
Oesophageal Diseases

Stephen Wilkinson
Derriford Hospital
Plymouth,
UK

A member of the Hodder Headline Group
LONDON
Copublished in the USA by
Oxford University Press, Inc., New York

First published in Great Britain in 1998
Reprinted in 2000 by Arnold, a member of the Hodder Headline Group,
338 Euston Road, London NW1 3BH

http://www.arnoldpublishers.com

Co-published in the USA by
Oxford University Press Inc.,
198 Madison Avenue, New York, NY10016
Oxford is a registered trademark of Oxford University Press

British Library Cataloguing in Publication Data
A catalogue record for this book is available from the British Library

Library of Congress Cataloging-in-Publication Data
A catalog record for this book is available from the Library of Congress

ISBN 0 412 80910 9

2 3 4 5 6 7 8 9 10

Typeset in 10/12pt Palatino by Keyset Composition, Colchester
Printed in Great Britain by St Edmundsbury Press and bound by MPG Books Ltd

What do you think about this book? Or any other Arnold title?
Please send your comments to feedback.arnold@hodder.co.uk

Contents

Preface

Oesophageal diseases, particularly gastro-oesophageal reflux, are extremely common. Nearly 10% of the population seek medical advice for reflux at some time in their lives. Furthermore, adenocarcinoma of the oesophagus, a consequence of gastro-oesophageal reflux, has been reported to be increasing in incidence more rapidly than any other malignancy in the Western world.

I make no apology for half of the text being devoted to gastro-oesophageal reflux. This is entirely appropriate considering the amount of time a practising gastroenterologist is involved in managing reflux and its many complications. Relatively little space is given to details of surgical management, emphasis being placed on the physician's role in selecting patients for surgery and managing subsequent complications. I have made every effort at least to mention most oesophageal diseases encountered in the Western world, but rare conditions are inevitably covered briefly, but hopefully succinctly. Subjects more often within the practice of otolaryngorhinologists are given only brief mention. Oesophageal varices are not included as this subject is more appropriate to a hepatological text. Oesophageal diseases in children are also omitted.

Like most sub-specialties within gastroenterology, oesophagology is multidisciplinary, but this book is written primarily for physicians. It is hoped that gastroenterologists in training will find it particularly useful. Surgeons, histopathologists and radiologists might also benefit from a physician's viewpoint.

I offer my warmest thanks to my colleagues with whom I worked during my previous appointment in Gloucester, particularly Michael Gear, Neil Shepherd, Ian Donald, Gary Ford and Stephen Gore, who all helped and encouraged me into the sub-specialty of oesophagology.

Stephen Wilkinson
Plymouth

1

Gastro-oesophageal reflux – prevalence, natural history, symptoms and diagnosis

Gastro-oesophageal reflux (GOR) is one of the most prevalent clinical disorders in the Western world. In a recent survey of 2112 adults in the UK a quarter had experienced heartburn, the cardinal symptom of reflux, during the preceding year, while 6% experienced heartburn at least weekly [1]. The incidence of reflux rises rapidly after the age of 40 (Figure 1.1) [2].

The incidence of endoscopic oesophagitis, a manifestation of GOR, has shown a substantial rise in recent decades. In one survey this increased from 10/100 000 in 1963 to 139/100 000 in 1980 [3] and more than quadrupled between 1977 and 1987 in another [4]. Whether this is a true rise in incidence or a result of more patients with reflux being referred for endoscopy is unclear, but undoubtedly reflux oesophagitis is now the most commonly found abnormality at diagnostic endoscopy [4].

GOR is a normal physiological event. Healthy asymptomatic subjects show acid reflux into the oesophagus sufficient to lower the pH to 4 or less up to 4% of the time. Precisely when reflux becomes abnormal is difficult or impossible to define, particularly as the severity of symptoms shows only a poor correlation with either the degree of acid reflux or whether or not oesophageal mucosal damage has occurred [5,6].

The oesophageal mucosa appears to react to reflux in one of four ways:

- no damage;
- erosive/ulcerative oesophagitis;
- stricture formation;
- replacement with columnar-lined (Barrett's) mucosa, which has malignant potential.

The group of patients without mucosal damage is itself heterogeneous. Many are part of the spectrum of 'classical' GOR disease and show abnormal acid reflux on pH testing, together with a correlation with

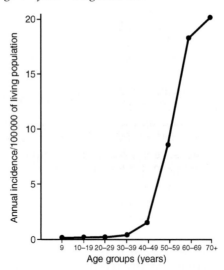

Figure 1.1   Illustrating the increasing incidence of gastro-oesophageal reflux with age. (Source: redrawn from reference 2, with permission of the publisher.)

symptoms. Two other groups are now also recognized and merit attention.

- **Acid-hypersensitive oesophagus.** These patients have typical symptoms of GOR but normal total 24-hour oesophageal acid exposure. However, the episodes of pain often coincide with acid reflux [7,8]. They are not only hypersensitive to acid, in that they have also been reported to show a lowered sensory threshold to balloon distension [8]. Long-term follow-up has shown they behave similarly to those with abnormal total acid exposure [9]. In fact, a minority of these patients with normal total acid exposure do show mild erosive oesophagitis [7].
- **Functional heartburn.** This is a condition in which the patients complain of reflux-like symptoms, but have entirely normal investigations: in particular there is no relationship between symptoms and episodes of acid reflux [10]. The heartburn may be postural, precipitated by food or provoked by stress/emotion and is more common during the day. It is often associated with upper abdominal discomfort, belching, nausea and early satiety. It is more common in females and may account for 20% of patients presenting with heartburn. It may be a variant of irritable bowel syndrome.

NATURAL HISTORY

There have been relatively few long-term serial studies of patients with GOR. Undoubtedly it is usually a chronic continuous or chronic relapsing disorder, but approximately one-third of patients may enter a sustained remission spontaneously [11–13]. More than 80% of patients with oesophagitis healed by omeprazole will relapse within 6 months after cessation of therapy [14].

In some patients the severity of mucosal damage increases with time. Five out of 33 patients with a previously normal mucosa developed endoscopic oesophagitis during a 3–6 month follow-up [11]. In a large retrospective study of 582 patients followed for a mean period of 6.5 years, 189 evolved to a more severe grade, 15 developed stricture and 55 columnar-lined oesophagus [15]. The natural history of the evolution of stricture and columnar-lined oesophagus is further discussed in Chapters 5 and 6 respectively. It is unknown whether patients with functional heartburn ever progress to oesophagitis, though some with acid hyper-sensitivity do [11].

SYMPTOMS

The cardinal symptom of GOR is a retrosternal burning pain, often radiating from the epigastrium into the throat. It is characteristically brought on by meals, lying flat or stooping forward. It is often accompanied by regurgitation. Odynophagia (painful swallowing), par-ticularly of hot, alcoholic or citrus drinks, is another common symptom. Patients with oesophagitis may complain of dysphagia in the absence of peptic stricture [16]. Female patients often give a history of heartburn during pregnancy.

Atypical symptoms of reflux include bleeding (either haematemesis, melaena or occult), epigastric or 'ulcer'-type pain, vomiting (N.B. oesophagitis may be **secondary** to vomiting), non-specific or even angina-like chest pain (Chapter 10).

Respiratory presentations of reflux have received much attention in recent years. These include hoarseness, globus, cough and asthma. However, the relationship with reflux and each of these has yet to be convincingly established (Chapter 7).

The oesophageal complications may be the first clinical manifestations of reflux. A peptic stricture will usually present as dysphagia. Barrett's oesophagus may present with symptoms from a carcinoma.

DIAGNOSIS OF UNCOMPLICATED GOR

Symptoms

The classical symptoms of food- or posture-related heartburn and regurgitation have a specificity for the diagnosis of gastro-oesophageal reflux of about 60%, but low sensitivity [17,18]. However, if either of these symptoms dominates the patient's complaints the specificity has been reported to rise to 90% [18].

Atypical presentations will require specific investigations to allow a confident diagnosis.

Endoscopy

Undoubtedly, endoscopy is the diagnostic test most widely used in the evaluation of patients with suspected gastro-oesophageal reflux. The earliest lesion is a discrete, often slightly depressed red area, usually with a whitish exudate, presumably secondary to acid–peptic erosion. These are situated just proximal to and usually in continuity with the squamocolumnar junction, particularly on the crests of the longitudinal mucosal folds (Plate 1). In more severe cases these lesions are joined up, and in the most severe are circumferential (Plate 2). There are many grading systems to assess the severity of oesophagitis, the most commonly used being that described by Savary and Miller (Table 1.1) [19]. In this system Stage I refers to isolated lesions, Stage II to confluent lesions, and Stage III to circumferential lesions. Stage IV does not code for the severity of the oesophagitis, but for the presence of complications. This grading system does not take into account the longitudinal extent of mucosal damage. Some confusion has inevitably arisen from the fact that Savary and others have changed his original classification.

If exudate is present on the lesion the diagnosis is straightforward, but when there are red spots or streaks without exudate the appearances may have poor specificity for reflux. Of 47 patients investigated by Monnier and Savary [20], biopsy of the red spots or streaks revealed histological oesophagitis, as assessed by polymorph infiltrate, in only 19. In the remaining patients the histological findings were normal in 17, nine had columnar mucosa, one exhibited moderate dysplasia and one patient had carcinoma-*in-situ*. All patients with exudate appeared to have histological oesophagitis. In this study control biopsies were taken from areas that appeared to be normal at the same level of the oesophagus in which the red areas were seen. The authors concluded that biopsy of a focal red area is mandatory, especially if the lesion is devoid of exudate.

Table 1.1   Staging of oesophagitis (Savary and Miller [19])

Stage I	One or more non-confluent reddish lesions with exudate
Stage II	The erosive and exudative lesions are confluent without covering the entire circumference of the oesophagus
Stage III	Circumferential involvement by the erosive/exudative lesions
Stage IV	Complications including Barrett's metaplasia, deep ulcers, stricture and oesophageal shortening

Table 1.2 Staging of oesophagitis (Los Angeles classification [21])

Grade A	One or more mucosal breaks confined to the mucosal folds, each no longer than 5 mm
Grade B	At least one mucosal break more than 5 mm long confined to the mucosal folds, but not continuous between the tops of two mucosal folds
Grade C	At least one mucosal break continuous between the tops of two or more mucosal folds but not circumferential
Grade D	Circumferential mucosal break

A more recent classification has been proposed by an international group (the 'Los Angeles classification') [21]. Because of lack of uniformity in the description of the lesions characteristic of oesophagitis as erosions by some and ulcers by others they have introduced the term 'mucosal break'. This is defined as an area of slough or an area of erythema with a discrete demarcation from the adjacent or normal-looking mucosa. However, histological confirmation of a true break in the squamous epithelium has yet to be provided. Their classification is based on the extent of the breaks (Table 1.2), with complications being described separately.

Diffuse erythema is also used as a marker of oesophagitis in some classifications, but others regard it as non-specific and age-related, and it may be transient and non-inflammatory [22].

Interobserver variation between endoscopists in recognition of manifestations of reflux has been carefully assessed by Bytzer *et al.* [23]. Three experienced endoscopists assessed 150 patients with dyspeptic symptoms. Interobserver agreement on erosive lesions was excellent and comparable to agreement on gastric and duodenal ulcer. However, for focal or diffuse erythema, and friability (another putative marker used in some classifications of reflux), agreement was poor, with kappa values of 0.34–0.47 (0 = no agreement; 0–0.4 = poor agreement; 0.4–0.7 = acceptable agreement; 0.7–1.0 = good agreement; 1.0 = complete agreement; Table 1.3).

In the more recent study of Armstrong *et al.* [21] interobserver variation was assessed using still or video images. There was good agreement on the presence or absence of mucosal breaks (kappa values 0.81–0.84), but less good in assessing their extent. However, agreement between expert endoscopists on focal erythema, diffuse erythema and friability was better than in the study of Bytzer *et al.*

The sensitivity of endoscopy in the diagnosis of reflux is poor, with only about 50% of patients showing erosive or ulcerative changes [6,24]. The potential additional value of biopsies has therefore been evaluated by several groups. Ismail-Beigi *et al.* [25] have proposed that epithelial

Table 1.3   Interobserver variation in diagnosis of 'minimal oesophagitis' (Bytzer *et al.* [23]); kappa = 0.34–0.47 (0.68–0.79 for erosive oesophagitis)

	Observer I	Observer II	Observer III
Focal erythema	16	23	32
Diffuse erythema	3	4	3
Friability	1	5	6
Any of these	17	28	35

hyperplasia, as manifest by basal cell thickening and papillary elongation, is the earliest histological change in reflux disease. However, other studies have cast doubt on this conclusion. Seefeld *et al.* [26] and Collins *et al.* [27] could not confirm epithelial hyperplasia to be a manifestation of reflux, while Weinstein *et al.* [28] found biopsies from 17 of 19 asymptomatic subjects to show epithelial hyperplasia.

A new approach has been proposed by Clark *et al.* [29]. In patients with reflux they have found histological evidence of inflammation in biopsies taken from the columnar epithelium immediately distal to the squamocolumnar junction more frequently than in biopsies from the squamous epithelium immediately proximal. Furthermore the changes ('carditis') have been related to the severity of reflux as assessed by oesophageal acid exposure. Their view of sphincter incompetence is that this occurs in a distal–proximal direction, the result of which would be for inflammatory changes to initially affect the intrasphincteric columnar mucosa. Such findings, if confirmed, could substantially improve the sensitivity of endoscopy in the diagnosis of reflux. However, we have not been able to relate histological carditis to reflux, but only to inflammation elsewhere in the stomach and to *Helicobacter* infection [30].

Many patients with endoscopic oesophagitis have a sliding hiatus hernia [6], but when oesophagitis is absent a hernia should not be regarded as a reliable sign of reflux (pp. 13–15).

There are other possible endoscopic manifestations of GOR. An oesophagogastric sphincter that remains patulous throughout the procedure together with free reflux would seem likely to be a true manifestation of GOR [6], but intermittent reflux of gastric contents might be secondary to patient straining. A sentinel nodule at the squamocolumnar junction and thickened distal oesophageal epithelium have also been suggested as manifestations of reflux. An inflammatory pseudotumour has been described as a manifestation of reflux [31].

pH monitoring

Continuous ambulatory 24-hour oesophageal pH monitoring is undoubtedly the most sensitive and most specific test available for diagnosing and quantifying GOR, but does not assess the degree of mucosal damage. It allows an assessment of the correlation between episodes of reflux and the patient's symptoms. However, it is somewhat cumbersome and not always well tolerated by patients. It is now widely available in district general hospitals [32]. It is more fully discussed in Chapter 19.

Contrast radiography

The most commonly used contrast material for diagnostic studies of the upper alimentary tract is barium. Three radiological findings are of relevance to the diagnosis of reflux: the demonstration of reflux, radiological signs of oesophagitis and the occurrence of a hiatus hernia.

The value of the barium examination in demonstrating reflux varies widely in different reports. Ott [33] has reviewed 10 series comprising 587 patients. The examination detected reflux in only 204 (35%) of proven cases. Provocative measures such as increasing intra-abdominal pressure or the 'water siphon test' (demonstration of reflux of barium during water swallowing) may increase the sensitivity to 70% [34,35].

Contrast radiology has a sensitivity of only about 60% for detecting endoscopic oesophagitis [30]. The changes include mucosal and contour irregularity, longitudinal fold thickening, erosions, ulcers and strictures.

As already pointed out, the occurrence of a hiatus hernia should not be equated with GOR [36]. Most patients with a hernia do not have reflux. However, severe oesophagitis is unusual without a hernia.

In view of the widely differing results and their own experience one group has concluded: 'The sensitivity and specificity of barium radiology for abnormal degrees of acid reflux are insufficient for it to be worthwhile as a screening procedure' [37].

Summary

Although the patient's history can have high specificity for the diagnosis of GOR the sensitivity is low. Endoscopy, if abnormal, has extremely high specificity but, again, relatively poor sensitivity. pH monitoring undoubtedly has the highest specificity and sensitivity, but is least acceptable to patients. The role of contrast radiology remains uncertain. The appropriate use of history and investigations is discussed further in Chapters 3 and 19.

REFERENCES

1. Penston JG, Pounder RE. A survey of dyspepsia in Great Britain. *Aliment Pharmacol Ther* 1996; **10**: 83–89.

2. Brunnen PL, Karmody AM, Needham CD. Severe peptic oesophagitis. *Gut* 1969; **10**: 832–837.

3. Ollyo J-B, Monnier P, Fontolliet C, Savary M. The natural history, prevalence and incidence of reflux oesophagitis. *Gullet* 1993; **3**(Suppl): 3–10.

4. Gear MWL, Wilkinson SP. Open-access upper alimentary endoscopy. *Br J Hosp Med* 1989; **41**: 438–444.

5. DeMeester TR, Wang CI, Wernly JA *et al.* Technique, indications and clinical use of 24 hour esophageal pH monitoring. *J Thorac Cardiovasc Surg* 1980; **79**: 656–670.

6. Johansson K-E, Ask P, Boeryd B *et al.* Oesophagitis, signs of reflux and gastric acid secretion in patients with symptoms of gastro-oesophageal reflux disease. *Scand J Gastroenterol* 1986; **21**: 837–847.

7. Shi G, Bruley des Varannes S, Scarpignato C *et al.* Reflux related symptoms in patients with normal oesophageal exposure to acid. *Gut* 1995; **37**: 457–464.

8. Trimble KC, Pryde A, Heading RC. Lowered oesophageal sensory thresholds in patients with symptomatic but not excess gastro-oesophageal reflux: evidence for a spectrum of visceral sensitivity in GORD. *Gut* 1995; **37**: 7–12.

9. Trimble KC, Douglas S, Pryde A, Heading RC. Clinical characteristics and natural history of symptomatic but not excess gastroesophageal reflux. *Dig Dis Sci* 1995; **40**: 1098–1104.

10. Richter JE. Functional esophageal disorders. In: Drossman DA, ed. The Functional Gastrointestinal Disorders. Boston, MA: Little, Brown, 1994: pp 25–70.

11. Pace F, Santalucia F, Bianchi Porro G. Natural history of gastro-oesophageal reflux disease without oesophagitis. *Gut* 1991; **32**: 845–848.

12. Schindlebeck NE, Klauser AJ, Berghammer G *et al.* Three year follow up of patient with gastro-oesophageal reflux disease. *Gut* 1992; **33**: 1016–1019.

13. Isolauri J, Luostarinen M, Isolauri E *et al.* Natural course of gastroesophageal reflux disease: 17–22 year follow up of 60 patients. *Am J Gastroenterol* 1997; **92**: 37–41.

14. Hetzel DJ, Dent J, Reed WD *et al.* Healing and relapse of severe peptic esophagitis after treatment with omeprazole. *Gastroenterology* 1988; **95**: 903–912.

15. Brossard E, Monnier P, Ollyo J-B *et al.* Serious complications – stenosis, ulcer and Barrett's epithelium – develop in 21.6% of adults with erosive reflux esophagitis. *Gastroenterology* 1991; **100**: A36.

16. Dakkak M, Hoare RC, Maslin SC, Bennett JR. Oesophagitis is as important as oesophageal stricture diameter in determining dysphagia. *Gut* 1993; **34**: 152–155.

17. Johnsson F, Joelsson B, Gudmundsson K *et al.* Symptoms and endoscopic findings in the diagnosis of gastroesophageal reflux disease. *Scand J Gastroenterol* 1987; **22**: 714–718.
18. Klauser AG, Schindlbeck NE, Müller-Lissner SA. Symptoms in gastro-oesophageal reflux disease. *Lancet* 1990; **335**: 205–208.
19. Savary M, Miller G. *The Oesophagus. Handbook and Atlas of Endoscopy.* Glassamann: Solothurn, 1978.
20. Monnier P, Savary M. Contribution of endoscopy to gastro-oesophageal reflux disease. *Scand J Gastroenterol* 1984; **19**(Suppl 106): 26–45.
21. Armstrong D, Bennett JR, Blum AL *et al.* The endoscopic assessment of esophagitis: a progress report on observer agreement. *Gastroenterology* 1996; **111**: 85–92.
22. Armstrong D, Monnier P, Nicolet M *et al.* Endoscopic assessment of oesophagitis. *Gullet* 1991; **1**: 63–67.
23. Bytzer P, Havelund T, Hansen JM. Interobserver variation in the endoscopic diagnosis of reflux oesophagitis. *Scand J Gastroenterol* 1993; **28**: 119–125.
24. Behar J, Biancani P, Sheahan DG. Evaluation of esophageal tests in the diagnosis of reflux esophagitis. *Gastroenterology* 1976; **71**: 9–15.
25. Ismail-Beigi F, Horton PF, Pope CE. Histological consequences of gastroesophageal reflux in man. *Gastroenterology* 1970; **58**: 163–174.
26. Seefeld U, Krejs GJ, Siebenmann RE, Blum AL. Esophageal histology in gastroesophageal reflux. *Am J Dig Dis* 1977; **22**: 956–964.
27. Collins BJ, Elliott H, Sloane JM *et al.* Oesophageal histology in reflux oesophagitis. *J Clin Pathol* 1985; **38**: 1265–1272.
28. Weinstein WM, Bogoch ER, Bowes KL. The normal human esophageal mucosa: a histological reappraisal. *Gastroenterology* 1975; **68**: 40–44.
29. Clark GWB, Ireland AP, Chandrasoma P *et al.* Inflammation and metaplasia in the transitional epithelium of the gastroesophageal junction: a new marker for gastroesophageal reflux disease. *Gastroenterology* 1994; **106**: A63.
30. Dunlop S, Sherwood A, Wilkinson SP. Gastric carditis – a manifestation of gastro-oesophageal reflux or *Helicobacter* infection? *Gut* 1998; **42** (Suppl 1): A16.
31. Staples DC, Knodell RG, Johnson LF. Inflammatory pseudotumor of the esophagus. *Gastrointest Endosc* 1978; **24**: 175–176.
32. Donald IP, Ford GA, Wilkinson SP. Is 24-hour ambulatory oesophageal pH monitoring useful in a district general hospital? *Lancet* 1987; **i**: 89–91.
33. Ott DJ. Gastroesophageal reflux: what is the role of barium studies? *AJR* 1994; **162**: 627–629.
34. Sellar RJ, de Caestecker JS, Heading RC. Barium radiology: a sensitive test for gastro-oesophageal reflux. *Clin Radiol* 1987; **38**: 303–307.

35. Thompson JK, Koehler RE, Richter JE. Detection of gastroesophageal reflux: value of barium studies compared with 24-hour pH monitoring. *AJR* 1994; **162**: 621–626.
36. Ott DJ. Radiology of esophageal function and gastroesophageal reflux disease. In: *Investigations in Esophageal Disease*. Scarpignato C, Galmiche J-P, eds. Basle: S Karger, 1994: pp 27–70.
37. Johnston BT, Troshinsky MB, Castell JA, Castell DO. Comparison of barium radiology with esophageal pH monitoring in the diagnosis of gastroesophageal reflux disease. *Am J Gastroenterol* 1996; **91**: 1181–1185.

2

Gastro-oesophageal reflux – pathophysiology and pathogenesis

The occurrence of abnormal GOR together with any consequent tissue damage is a multifactorial process involving sphincter failure, poor clearance of refluxed material, toxicity of the refluxate to the oesophageal mucosa and impaired gastric emptying (Table 2.1). Although different factors may have differing roles in individual patients it is increasingly recognized that dysfunction of the lower oesophageal sphincter (LOS) is usually of paramount importance.

Table 2.1 Factors involved in the pathophysiology of gastro-oesophageal reflux disease

---

- Sphincter dysfunction
  - Transient lower oesophageal sphincter relaxations
  - Basal lower oesophageal sphincter pressure
  - Hiatus hernia
  - Flap valve
  - Sphincter length
  - Length of intra-abdominal oesophagus
  - Mucosal choke
  - Dietary factors, smoking
  - Drugs
  - Psychological factors
- Factors determining oesophageal damage
  - Sphincter dysfunction
  - Acid/pepsin
  - Impaired oesophageal clearance
  - Impaired gastric emptying
  - Mucosal resistance
  - *Helicobacter* infection (may be protective)

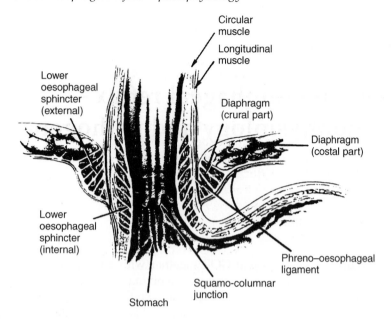

Figure 2.1 The lower oesophageal sphincter. (Source: redrawn from reference 1, with permission of the publisher.)

FACTORS DETERMINING ABNORMAL REFLUX

Sphincter dysfunction and role of hiatus hernia

The LOS is an anatomically complex structure some 4 cm in length (Figure 2.1). The internal sphincter is made up of the oesophageal smooth muscle and the muscle sling of the proximal stomach. The crural diaphragm constitutes the external sphincter. The distal oesophagus is attached to the diaphragm by the pheno-oesophageal ligament. Other factors contributing to sphincter function, which are largely self explanatory and will not therefore be discussed in detail, include the flap valve formed as a result of the angle between the oesophagus and the gastric cardia, the overall length of the LOS, the length of the intra-abdominal segment of the oesophagus and a mucosal choke formed by apposition of the collapsed oesophagus [1].

Basal LOS pressure may be very low in patients with GOR, but there is a large overlap with control subjects [2–4]. More subtle explanations have therefore been sought and provided, particularly by Dent and colleagues with the identification of transient lower oesophageal sphincter relaxations (TLOSRs).

Although it is well known that the LOS will transiently relax in response to swallowing, Dent and others have demonstrated sphincter relaxation in the absence of a preceding swallow and that these events may result in reflux (Figure 2.2) [5–7].

He has coined the term 'transient lower oesophageal sphincter relaxation'. Characteristically these are of longer duration (10–45 s) than swallow-induced relaxations (6–8 s). They are triggered by gaseous or food distension of the stomach and by pharyngeal stimulation. They are mediated by vagal activity [7] and endogenous cholecystokinin [8]. The frequency of TLOSRs is reduced, but not abolished, in the supine posture and during deep sleep. There is also complete selective inhibition of the crural diaphragm during TLOSR, in contrast to swallow-induced sphincter relaxation, which results in only partial crural inhibition [7]. As the events during a TLOSR are identical to those observed with belching, the normal physiological mechanism whereby the stomach vents swallowed air, a TLOSR may be regarded as a variant of the belch reflex.

By using combined oesophageal pH/manometry measurements in both stationary and ambulant settings Dent's group have shown that more than 80% of reflux episodes in healthy control subjects are a result of TLOSRs, most of the others being swallow-related [5,9]. In patients, TLOSRs accounted for two-thirds of the episodes of recorded reflux, the remainder being due to free reflux through a sphincter with low basal pressure, events raising intra-abdominal pressure or swallowing in roughly equal numbers [6,10]. Compared with control subjects patients have more frequent episodes of TLOSRs and these are more likely to be associated with reflux. Dent's studies have repeatedly shown that the non-TLOSR mechanisms are more frequent causes of reflux in patients with more severe oesophagitis.

Even though TLOSRs are suppressed in the supine posture these remain the main mechanism for supine reflux [11]. At night the majority of reflux episodes also occur as a result of TLOSRs, mostly during arousal [12]. However, other mechanisms for reflux may occur during sleep, e.g. through a patulous sphincter.

In view of the importance of the crura of the diaphragm as part of the lower oesophageal sphincter, a sliding hiatus hernia would be expected to disrupt the overall sphincter mechanism (Figures 2.1 and 14.1a). This might be particularly important in reflux secondary to increased intra-abdominal pressure [13].

A hernia may have an accessory role in some patients by a mechanism other than disrupting the sphincter. Mittal *et al.* [14] have shown that acid, after clearance from the oesophagus, may remain trapped in the hernia sack and so be available for reflux during the next swallow-induced LOS relaxation.

Although a hernia is more commonly found in patients with GOR, it is inappropriate to use the term as being synonymous with reflux as the relationship is inconsistent (Chapter 1). Bennett [15] has suggested: 'It

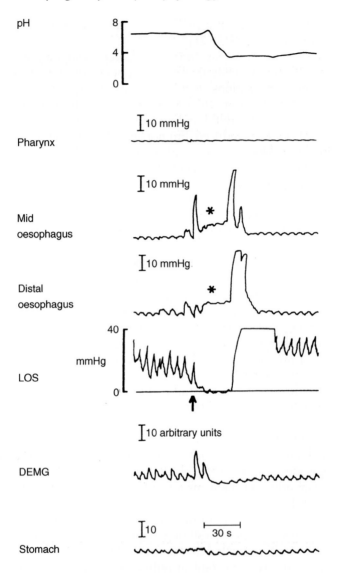

Figure 2.2 A spontaneous transient lower oesophageal sphincter (LOS) relaxation (arrow). This is followed by acid reflux into the oesophagus (channel pH). Note that there is no preceding oesophageal peristaltic wave. DEMG = diaphragm electomyelogram. (Source: redrawn from reference 7, with permission of the publisher.)

would be desirable if the term "hiatus hernia" ceased to be used as a diagnostic label in patients with reflux symptoms'.

An alternative view to the relationship between GOR and a hiatus hernia has been considered by Paterson and Kolyn. [16]. Acid installation into the oesophagus of the opossum resulted in longitudinal shortening, suggesting that acid reflux could cause a sliding hiatus hernia. Thus a vicious cycle could develop in some patients. TLOSR-induced reflux might lead to oesophageal shortening, with disruption of the LOS and worsening reflux [1].

Dietary factors and drugs

Fat, chocolate, alcohol and smoking may all promote reflux, as may various drugs. The latter include theophylline, nitrates, calcium-channel blockers and progestogens. These are all more fully discussed in Chapter 3.

Psychological factors

The importance of psychological factors, particularly stress, has received little attention until recently. A survey in North America found that 64% of those questioned who suffered heartburn noted that their symptoms were exacerbated by stress [17]. Compared with healthy control subjects, patients with GOR disease have increased anxiety, obsessionality, pessimism, alimentary susceptibility, depression, hassles perceived with greater intensity, and poor social support [18], but in one study the difference in psychological profile compared with controls was due to a subset of patients that constituted 30% of the total series [19].

Although stress can increase susceptibility to symptoms [20,21] this is not the only explanation. Relaxation therapy has been shown to reduce oesophageal acid exposure in a group of patients with GOR [22].

FACTORS DETERMINING OESOPHAGEAL DAMAGE

Duration of oesophageal acid exposure/acid clearance/saliva/ oesophageal and gastric dysmotility

Gastric acid is undoubtedly the most important component of refluxate that damages the oesophageal mucosa. This is most convincingly demonstrated by the fact that potent acid suppression by a proton-pump inhibitor will render most patients symptom-free and completely heal their oesophagitis (Chapter 3). GOR is not usually associated with increased acid output [23] but, when acid secretion is increased, as in

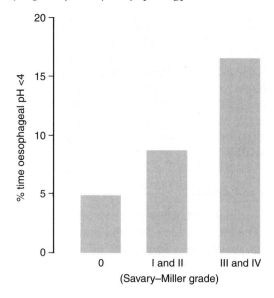

Figure 2.3   Relationship of oesophageal acid exposure to severity of endoscopic oesophagitis. (Source: adapted from reference 25, with permission of the publisher.)

Zollinger–Ellison syndrome, oesophagitis is common [24]. Pepsin is an additional aggressive factor and requires an acid medium to be active [23].

The severity of oesophagitis is related to the total time of distal oesophageal acid exposure (Figure 2.3) [25–27].

On the basis of continuous oesophageal pH recordings several groups have suggested nocturnal/supine reflux to be more injurious [25,28,29], but this has not been confirmed by others [27]. The latter group have shown a better correlation between endoscopic damage and reflux after the evening meal.

Acid clearance is dependent upon not only effective oesophageal peristalsis, but also the neutralizing effect of swallowed saliva [30]. Saliva also contains other beneficial constituents, including epidermal growth factor [31].

Primary peristalsis has been shown by 24-hour pH/motility studies to be the main peristaltic mechanism for clearing refluxate from the oesophagus [32]. It has the additional advantage over secondary peristalsis that saliva will also be delivered to the oesophagus. Secondary peristalsis will reduce the volume of the refluxate but will not affect pH until it has been entirely cleared. As primary peristalsis does not occur during sleep, reflux can therefore result in prolonged oesophageal acid

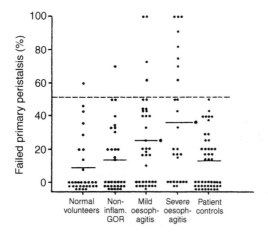

Figure 2.4 Relationship of rate of failed wet-swallow-induced primary peristalsis to severity of oesophagitis. (Source: redrawn from reference 4, with permission of the publisher.)

exposure unless there is arousal, resulting in additional swallowing and primary peristalsis [33].

It has long been recognized that primary peristalsis may be deficient with GOR. In patients with oesophagitis Olsen and Schlegel [34] demonstrated low-amplitude peristalsis in 37%, peristaltic failure in 8% and motor incoordination in 32%. These findings have been confirmed in many more recent studies (Figure 2.4) [4]. Certainly, they may be relevant to impaired clearance of refluxate.

Other motility disorders described include failed secondary peristalsis [35] and diminished oesophageal contractile force [36].

All the above oesophageal motility abnormalities are more marked in patients with the most severe oesophagitis.

The motility disorders of GOR are not confined to the oesophagus. Delayed gastric emptying has been repeatedly demonstrated and would inevitably have an adverse effect on GOR, particularly with respect to the volume of refluxate [37]. Furthermore, it is predictable that the associated gastric distension will provoke TLOSRs.

Reflux of duodenal contents

Bile acids, particularly in an acid medium, may cause oesophageal mucosal damage [38]. Duodenogastro-oesophageal (DGOR) might therefore be a further pathogenic factor in reflux disease. This concept has been given credence by 24-hour ambulatory DGOR measurements using a bilirubin-detecting fibreoptic probe (Bilitec). Vaezi and Richter. [39] have confirmed DGOR to occur with increasing severity across the spectrum of

GOR disease from controls to uncomplicated reflux to complicated reflux. The results paralleled those for acid reflux. Marshall *et al.* [40], using the same technique, have shown DGOR alone to be an unusual cause of symptoms.

Resistance of oesophageal mucosa to damage by refluxate

Although patients with the greatest oesophageal acid exposure tend to have the most severe mucosal damage, the large overlap between different groups points to the possibility of local mucosal factors being of importance in resisting reflux-induced damage. Acid perfusion of the oesophagus results in a marked increase in mucosal bicarbonate, which could have an important effect on mucosal defence [41]. Local mucus secretion might also be important [42].

Helicobacter pylori infection

Gastric infection with *Helicobacter pylori* does not appear to have any direct role in the pathogenesis of GOR disease [43,44]. However, of more than 200 patients with duodenal ulcer who were cured of the infection reflux oesophagitis emerged in 26% [45,46]. This was associated with greater gastric acid production after the infection had been eradicated, possibly because these patients had more severe inflammation of the body of the stomach, the site of acid production, before cure. Thus *Helicobacter* infection may 'protect' some individuals from developing GOR disease.

SUMMARY OF PATTERNS OF ABNORMAL REFLUX AND MOTILITY CHANGES

Considering patterns of reflux, sphincteric and motility disturbances, and the severity of the mucosal damage a spectrum emerges (Table 2.2). The mildest disease is characterized by upright reflux, reflux episodes largely due to TLOSRs, good basal sphincter tone, good propagated oesophageal peristalsis and contractile function, and no oesophagitis. At the other end of the spectrum patients with the most severe mucosal disease have combined upright/supine reflux, reflux episodes due to both TLOSRs and other mechanisms, poor or even absent basal sphincter pressure and impaired oesophageal peristalsis. However, it is to be emphasized that these extremes bear little relationship to the patient's symptoms [26,47].

Looking at these two groups of patients raises a number of questions.

Table 2.2 Spectrum of major abnormalities in gastro-oesophageal reflux disease

- 'Mild' disease
  - No oesophagitis
  - Upright reflux
  - Reflux due to TLOSRs
  - Good basal sphincter tone
  - Good oesophageal peristalsis
- 'Severe' disease
  - Erosive oesophagitis and other complications
  - Upright and supine reflux
  - Reflux due to TLOSRs and other mechanisms
  - Poor basal sphincter tone
  - Poor oesophageal clearance

- **Does mild disease progress to severe disease?** The limited published serial studies available suggest that this may occur but is unusual (Chapter 1). Most patients with severe disease have the range of abnormalities on presentation, which is often soon after the onset of symptoms.
- **Can mucosal damage from reflux cause a reduced sphincter pressure and impaired motility?** Several studies have investigated basal sphincter pressure, oesophageal peristaltic activity and acid exposure after healing of oesophagitis with omeprazole, but failed to find any improvement [48–51]. However, these studies are relatively short-term, at most after only 6 months of treatment. It is not inconceivable that it might take much longer for these functions to improve. In one short-term study, healing of the oesophagitis resulted in an improvement in oesophageal contractile function [52]. It must therefore be concluded that the current limited data favour the view that the motility disturbances accompanying oesophagitis are not secondary to mucosal damage, are more likely to be primary manifestations of the disease, and that they would themselves result in an accentuation of mucosal damage.

ROLE OF VAGAL NERVE DYSFUNCTION

Several groups have suggested that abnormalities of vagal function underlie the pathogenesis of GOR [7,53]. Mention has already been made of the importance of vagal function in TLOSRs. It is also possible that the severe motility disturbances in the patients with the most severe mucosal disease could also have a similar mechanism. Abnormal vagal function and reflexes have been demonstrated in patients with oesophagitis [53,54].

GASTRO-OESOPHAGEAL REFLUX AND OESOPHAGITIS FOLLOWING PARTIAL OR TOTAL GASTRECTOMY AND IN PATIENTS WITH PERNICIOUS ANAEMIA

GOR and oesophagitis may occur following proximal or distal partial gastrectomy, or total gastrectomy, or be associated with pernicious anaemia [55–58]. As these conditions are associated with hypochlorhydria or achlorhydria, a role for non-acid reflux, in particular duodenogastro-oesophageal reflux, has been proposed.

In one study 32 patients who had undergone distal partial gastrectomy (Billroth I or Billroth II) and who had symptoms suggestive of gastro-oesophageal reflux were evaluated for both acid reflux (by pH monitoring) and DGOR (by Bilitec). Although symptoms often occurred with DGOR alone, oesophagitis was only found when there was also evidence for abnormal acid reflux [58].

Oesophagitis is almost invariable following proximal gastrectomy carried out for carcinoma of the gastric cardia, and is usually related to increased acid reflux [57].

The occurrence of oesophagitis following total gastrectomy is much less common [57] but is well documented [54] and can even progress to columnar (Barrett's) metaplasia with adenocarcinoma [59]. Non-acid reflux must be implicated in the pathogenesis and also when oesophagitis occurs in association with pernicious anaemia [56].

REFERENCES

1. Mittal RK, Balaban DH. The esophagogastric junction. *N Engl J Med* 1997; **336**: 924–932.
2. Behar J, Biancana P, Sheahan DG. Evaluation of esophageal tests in the diagnosis of reflux esophagitis. *Gastroenterology* 1976; **71**: 9–15.
3. Stanciu C, Hoare RC, Bennett JR. Correlation between manometric and pH tests for gastro-oesophageal reflux. *Gut* 1977; **18**: 536–540.
4. Kahrilas PJ, Dodds WJ, Hogan WJ *et al*. Esophageal peristaltic dysfunction in peptic esophagitis. *Gastroenterology* 1986; **91**: 897–904.
5. Dent J, Dodds WJ, Friedman RH *et al*. Mechanism of gastroesophageal reflux in recumbent asymptomatic human subjects. *J Clin Invest* 1980; **65**: 256–267.
6. Dodds WJ, Dent J, Hogan WJ *et al*. Mechanisms of gastroesophageal

reflux in patients with reflux esophagitis. *N Engl J Med* 1982; **307**: 1547–1552.

7. Mittal RK, Holloway RH, Penagini R *et al.* Transient lower esophageal sphincter relaxation. *Gastroenterology* 1995; **109**: 601–610.

8. Boulant J, Mathieu S, D'Amato M *et al.* Cholecystokinin in transient lower oesophageal sphincter relaxation due to gastric distension in humans. *Gut* 1997; **40**: 575–581.

9. Schoeman MN, Tippett MD, Akkermans LMA *et al.* Mechanisms of gastroesophageal reflux in ambulant healthy human subjects. *Gastroenterology* 1995; **108**: 83–91.

10. Penagini R, Schoeman MN, Holloway RH *et al.* Mechanisms of gastroesophageal reflux in ambulant patients with reflux esophagitis. *Gastroenterology* 1994; **106**: A159.

11. Freidin N, Mittal RK, McCallum RW. Does body posture affect the incidence and mechanism of gastro-oesophageal reflux? *Gut* 1991; **32**: 133–136.

12. Freidin N, Fisher MJ, Taylor W *et al.* Sleep and nocturnal acid reflux in normal subjects and patients with reflux oesophagitis. *Gut* 1991; **32**: 1275–1279.

13. Sloan S, Rademaker AW, Kahrilas PJ. Determinance of gastroesophageal junction incompetence: hiatal hernia, lower esophageal sphincter, or both? *Ann Intern Med* 1992; **117**: 977–982.

14. Mittal RK, Lange RC, McCallum RW. Identification and mechanism of delayed oesophageal acid clearance in subjects with hiatal hernia. *Gastroenterology* 1987; **92**: 130–135.

15. Bennett JR. Gastro-oesophageal reflux disease. In: Bouchier IAD, Allan RN, Hodgson HJF, Keighley MRB, eds. *Gastroenterology – Clinical Science and Practice.* 2nd ed. Philadelphia, PA: WB Saunders, 1993: p 83.

16. Paterson WG, Kolyn DM. Esophageal shortening induced by short-term intraluminal acid perfusion in opossum: a cause for hiatus hernia? *Gastroenterology* 1994; **107**: 1736–1740.

17. Gallup. *Gallup Survey of Heartburn Across America.* Princeton, NJ: Gallup Organization, 1988.

18. Johnston BT, Lewis SA, Love AHG. Psychological factors in gastro-oesophageal reflux disease. *Gut* 1995; **36**: 481–482.

19. Baker LH, Lieberman D, Oehlke M. Psychological distress in patients with gastroesophageal reflux disease. *Am J Gastroenterol* 1995; **90**: 1797–1803.

20. Bradley LA, Richter JE, Pulliam TJ *et al.* Psychological factors influence the relationship between stress and reports of gastroesophageal reflux. *Am J Gastroenterol* 1993; **88**: 11–19.

21. Johnston BT, Lewis SA, Collins JSA *et al.* Acid perception in gastro-oesophageal reflux disease is dependent on psychosocial

factors. *Scand J Gastroenterol* 1995; **30**: 1–5.
22. McDonald-Haile J, Bradley LA, Bailey MA *et al.* Relaxation training reduces symptom reports and acid exposure in patients with gastroesophageal reflux disease. *Gastroenterology* 1994; **107**: 61–69.
23. Hirschowitz BI. A critical analysis, with appropriate controls, of gastric acid and pepsin secretion in clinical esophagitis. *Gastroenterology* 1991; **101**: 1149–1158.
24. Miller LS, Vinayek R, Frucht H *et al.* Reflux esophagitis in patients with Zollinger–Ellison syndrome. *Gastroenterology* 1990; **98**: 341–345.
25. Johansson KE, Ask P, Boeryd B *et al.* Esophagitis, signs of reflux and gastric acid secretion in patients with symptoms of gastro-oesophageal reflux disease. *Scand J Gastroenterol* 1986; **21**: 837–847.
26. Johnsson F, Joelsson B, Gudmundsson K, Greiff L. Symptoms and endoscopic findings in the diagnosis of gastroesophageal reflux disease. *Scand J Gastroenterol* 1987; **22**: 714–718.
27. de Caestecker JS, Blackwell JN, Pryde A, Heading RC. Daytime gastro-oesophageal reflux is important in oesophagitis. *Gut* 1987; **28**: 519–526.
28. Robertson D, Aldersley M, Shepherd H, Smith CL. Patterns of acid reflux in complicated oesophagitis. *Gut* 1987; **28**: 1484–1488.
29. Orr WC, Allen ML, Robinson M. The pattern of nocturnal and diurnal esophageal acid exposure in the pathogenesis of erosive mucosal damage. *Am J Gastroenterol* 1994; **89**: 509–512.
30. Helm JF, Dodds WJ, Hogan WJ. Salivary response to esophageal acid in normal subjects and patients with reflux esophagitis. *Gastroenterology* 1987; **93**: 1393–1397.
31. Sarosiek J, Scheurich J, Marcinkiewicz M, McCallum RW. Enhancement of salivary esophagoprotection: rationale for a physiological approach to gastroesophageal reflux disease. *Gastroenterology* 1996; **110**: 675–681.
32. Anggiansah A, Taylor G, Bright N *et al.* Primary peristalsis is the major acid clearance mechanism in reflux patients. *Gut* 1994; **35**: 1536–1542.
33. Orr WC, Johnson LF, Robinson MG. Effect of sleep on swallowing, esophageal peristalsis and acid clearance. *Gastroenterology* 1984; **86**: 814–819.
34. Olsen AM, Schlegel JF. Motility disturbances caused by esophagitis. *J Thorac Cardiovasc Surg* 1965; **50**: 607–612.
35. Schoeman MN, Holloway RH. Integrity and characteristics of secondary oesophageal peristalsis in patients with gastro-oesophageal reflux disease. *Gut* 1995; **36**: 499–504.
36. Williams D, Thompson DG, Marples M *et al.* Identification of an abnormal esophageal clearance response to intraluminal distension in patients with esophagitis. *Gastroenterology* 1992; **103**: 943–953.

37. Richter JE. Delayed gastric emptying in reflux patients: to be or not to be? *Am J Gastroenterol* 1997; **92**: 1077–1078.
38. Vaezi MF, Singh S, Richter JE. Role of acid in duodenogastric reflux in esophageal mucosal injury: a review of animal and human studies. *Gastroenterology* 1995; **108**: 1897–1907.
39. Vaezi MF, Richter JE. Role of acid and duodenogastroesophageal reflux in gastroesophageal reflux disease. *Gastroenterology* 1996; **111**: 1192–1199.
40. Marshall REK, Anggiansah A, Owen WA, Owen WJ. The relationship between acid and bile reflux and symptoms in gastro-oesophageal reflux disease. *Gut* 1997; **40**: 182–187.
41. Brown CM, Rees WDW. Review article: Factors protecting the oesophagus against acid-mediated injury. *Aliment Pharmacol Ther* 1995; **9**: 251–262.
42. Namiot Z, Sarosiek J, Rourk RM *et al.* Human esophageal secretion: mucosal response to luminal acid and pepsin. *Gastroenterology* 1994; **106**: 973–981.
43. Newton M, Bryan R, Burnham WR, Kamm MA. Evaluation of *Helicobacter pylori* in reflux oesophagitis and Barrett's oesophagus. *Gut* 1997; **40**: 9–13.
44. Csendes A, Smok G, Cerda G *et al.* Prevalence of *Helicobacter pylori* infection in 190 controlled subjects and in 236 patients with gastroesophageal reflux, erosive esophagitis or Barrett's esophagus. *Dis Esoph* 1997; **10**: 38–42.
45. Labenz J, Blum AL, Bayerdörffer E *et al.* Curing *Helicobacter pylori* infection in patients with duodenal ulcer may provoke reflux esophagitis. *Gastroenterology* 1997; **112**: 1442–1447.
46. Labenz J, Tillenburg B, Peitz U *et al.* Effect of omeprazole one year after cure of *Helicobacter pylori* infection in duodenal ulcer patients. *Am J Gastroenterol* 1997; **92**: 576–581.
46a.Malfertheiner P, Veldhuyzen van Zanten S, Dent J *et al.* Does cure of *Helicobacter pylori* infection induce heartburn? *Gastroenterology* 1998; **114**; A598.
46b.Talley N J, Janssens J, Lauritsen K *et al.* No increase in reflux symptoms or esophagitis in patients with non-ulcer dyspepsia 12 months after *Helicobacter pylori* eradication. A randomized double-blind placebo controlled trial. *Gastroenterology* 1998; **114**: A598.
47. Knill-Jones RP, Card WI, Crean GP *et al.* The symptoms of gastro-oesophageal reflux and of oesophagitis. *Scand J Gastroenterol* 1984; **19**(Suppl 106): 72–76.
48. Singh P, Adamopoulos A, Taylor RH, Colin-Jones DG. Oesophageal motor function before and after healing of oesophagitis. *Gut* 1992; **33**: 1590–1596.
49. Singh P, Taylor RH, Colin-Jones DG. Prolonged remission of

oesophagitis does not alter the magnitude of oesophageal acid exposure. *Scand J Gastroenterol* 1994; **29**: 11–16.

50. Howard JM, Reynolds RPE, Frei JV *et al*. Macroscopic healing of esophagitis does not improve esophageal motility. *Dig Dis Sci* 1994; **39**: 648–654.

51. Timmer R, Breumelhof R, Nadorp JHSM, Smout AJPM. Oesophageal motility and gastro-oesophageal reflux before and after healing of reflux oesophagitis. A study using 24 hour ambulatory pH and pressure monitoring. *Gut* 1994; **35**: 1519–1522.

52. Williams D, Thompson DG, Heggie L *et al*. Esophageal clearance function following treatment of esophagitis. *Gastroenterology* 1994; **106**: 108–116.

53. Ogilvie AL, James PD, Atkinson M. Impairment of vagal function in reflux oesophagitis. *Q J Med* 1985; **54**: 61–74.

54. Chakraborty TK, Ogilvie AL, Heading RC, Ewing DJ. Abnormal cardiovascular reflexes in patients with gastro-oesophageal reflux. *Gut* 1989; **30**: 46–49.

55. Helsingen N. Oesophagitis following total gastrectomy. A follow-up study on nine patients five years or more after operation. *Acta Chir Scand* 1959; **118**: 190–202.

56. Palmer ED. Subacute erosive ('peptic') esophagitis associated with achlorhydria. *N Engl J Med* 1960; **262**: 927–929.

57. Shu C-P, Chen C-Y, Hsieh Y-H *et al*. Esophageal reflux after total or proximal gastrectomy in patients with adenocarcinoma of the gastric cardia. *Am J Gastroenterol* 1997; **92**: 1347–1350.

58. Vaezi MF, Richter JE. Contribution of acid and duodenogastro-oesophageal reflux to oesophageal mucosal injury and symptoms in partial gastrectomy patients. *Gut* 1997; **41**: 297–302.

59. Nishimaki T, Watanabe K, Suzuki T *et al*. Early esophageal adenocarcinoma arising in a short segment of Barrett's mucosa after total gastrectomy. *Am J Gastroenterol* 1996; **91**: 1856–1857.

3

Gastro-oesophageal reflux – medical management

The obvious aim of treatment of GOR is to improve or abolish symptoms. More contentious is whether or not it is necessary to keep the mucosa healed. Undoubtedly some patients with mild or no oesophagitis do progress with time to more severe disease or the complications of stricture or Barrett's oesophagus, but this appears to be relatively unusual (Chapter 1). Although it seems likely that effective treatment will prevent progression, long-term confirmatory randomized studies have yet to be carried out.

LIFE-STYLE MODIFICATIONS

With the availability of the highly effective proton-pump inhibitors for the treatment of GOR, simple and effective life-style modifications are easily forgotten. It is common sense that large meals taken near to bedtime might provoke nocturnal reflux. Patients are usually aware of this and should leave at least 2 hours after a meal before retiring. Fat ingestion is particularly deleterious: it reduces lower oesophageal sphincter pressure and increases oesophageal acid exposure [1,2]. Obese patients are usually advised to lose weight. However, recent studies have questioned whether weight loss *per se* reduces reflux [3,4]. It may be the reduced fat intake of a weight-reducing diet that is actually beneficial [5]. Other foods and drinks known to exacerbate reflux include, particularly, chocolate [2,6] and alcohol [7]. Coffee, but not tea, may induce reflux, an effect partially reversed by decaffeination [8]. Smoking may undoubtedly impair sphincter function and promote reflux [9,10], but the author has never witnessed an improvement in reflux symptoms as a result of a patient giving up smoking.

Elevation of the head of the bed for night-time refluxers, though sometimes difficult for the patient and his/her spouse to live with, may promote healing of oesophagitis [11,12]. Tightly fitting clothes around the abdomen should be avoided.

Some drugs impair sphincter function including theophylline, nitrates, calcium-channel blockers and progestogens. Their prescription may therefore have to be modified.

Stress may be a particularly important factor to address. Two-thirds of patients with heartburn report that their symptoms are much worse at times of stress [13]. Effective stress management can reduce total oesophageal acid exposure [14].

DRUGS

Antacids

Self-prescribed antacids, often in combination with alginic acid, are probably the most widely used medication for the treatment of GOR. They usually induce rapid symptom relief. Some placebo-controlled trials have shown evidence for objective benefits and have been reviewed by Sontag [15].

Motility drugs

To improve the underlying dysmotility of GOR is a logical approach to treatment. This would entail reducing transient lower oesophageal sphincter relaxations, and improving basal sphincter tone, oesophageal motility and gastric emptying when these are defective. Attempts to reduce transient lower oesophageal sphincter relaxations, the mechanism underlying most episodes of abnormal reflux, are discussed later in this chapter.

Metoclopramide and domperidone are the longest established drugs in this group in the UK. Controlled trials have shown only minimal objective evidence of benefit (reviewed by Ramirez and Richter [16]). Use of metoclopramide is frequently complicated by extrapyramidal side-effects. Domperidone is better tolerated, the main side-effect being hyperprolactinaemia and its consequences.

Bethanechol is a cholinergic agonist that has been widely used in the USA. Limited data suggest it to be about as effective as H_2-receptor antagonists in terms of both symptom relief and healing of oesophagitis [16]. Cholinergic side-effects may limit its use.

Cisapride acts by increasing availability of acetylcholine from postganglionic nerve endings in the myenteric plexus. It may increase basal sphincter pressure, improve the amplitude of oesophageal contraction and accelerate gastric emptying [16,17]. However, in patients the mechanism whereby it reduces oesophageal acid exposure appears to be by increasing the number of oesophageal contractions during reflux episodes rather than by any effect on sphincter pressure [18]. A potential additional beneficial effect of cisapride is that it may substantially increase salivary volume, including bicarbonate and epidermal growth factor secretion [19]. Side-effects are relatively unusual, the most common being abdominal cramp and diarrhoea. Recommended doses are from 10 mg twice daily to 20 mg three times daily.

For both symptom relief and healing of oesophagitis cisapride has been shown to be superior to placebo and of similar efficacy to H_2-receptor antagonists [16,20]. The combination of cisapride with an H_2-receptor antagonist is more effective than either drug alone [21,22].

Three European placebo-controlled trials have shown cisapride to be superior to placebo in maintaining remission in healed oesophagitis [23–25], but it is much less effective than omeprazole [26]. Approximately 70% of patients with healed grade I oesophagitis and 55% of those with healed grade II oesophagitis will be maintained in remission at 1 year. It is less effective for patients whose symptoms were recalcitrant or who had severe oesophagitis [27].

H_2-receptor antagonists

Although H_2-receptor antagonists had a huge impact on the management of peptic ulcer disease, their use in GOR, in terms of both symptomatic relief and healing, has been disappointing. There are various reasons for this.

● Total acid suppression is inadequate.
● They do not inhibit meal-induced acid secretion.
● Tolerance rapidly develops.

A greater degree of acid suppression is necessary for healing of oesophagitis than peptic ulcer. Bell and others [28] have shown by meta-analysis that if intragastric acidity is maintained at pH < 4 for 20–22 hours per day for 8 weeks 90% of patients will heal. This is not achievable by conventional doses of H_2-receptor antagonists. Meal-induced acid secretion is important in gastro-oesophageal reflux [29] and is not inhibited by H_2-receptor antagonists [30].

Several studies have shown that tolerance to the acid suppressing effect of H_2-receptor antagonists may occur in as little as 2 weeks (Figure 3.1) [31–33]. This does not occur with proton-pump inhibitors.

Sontag [15] has analysed the published trials of the use of H_2-receptor antagonists in the treatment of GOR and has concluded that symptom relief is achieved in about half, but when compared with placebo, complete healing is rare.

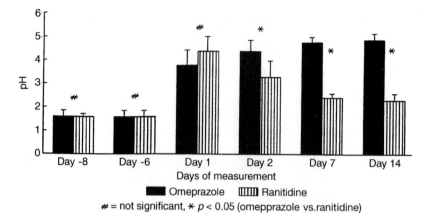

Figure 3.1 Development of tolerance to H_2-receptor antagonist after only 2 weeks of treatment. Vertical axis shows median 24-hour intragastric pH. (Source: redrawn from reference 33, with permission of the publisher.)

Proton-pump inhibitors

Proton-pump inhibitors (PPIs), particularly omeprazole, have transformed the medical management of GOR. They inhibit the K^+–H^+ ATPase on the secretory side of the gastric parietal cell, the final common pathway of acid secretion. Both basal and stimulated acid secretion are therefore inhibited. Omeprazole was the first such drug to be introduced. More recently, lansoprazole and pantoprazole have become available. They are generally very well tolerated, but about 5% of patients experience side-effects, in particular headache, nausea and diarrhoea, which may limit their use.

Most randomized controlled trials have been restricted to patients with endoscopic oesophagitis. A few trials of GOR without oesophagitis, acid-sensitive oesophagus and functional heartburn have now also been carried out.

For the treatment of oesophagitis, results from controlled trials have been reviewed by Sontag [15] and Bell and Hunt [34]. Sontag has analysed nine trials of the use of omeprazole 20–40 mg daily, involving more than 1300 patients, most studies randomizing patients against H_2-receptor antagonists. There was consistent therapeutic gain in both symptom relief and endoscopic healing. Most patients achieved complete symptom relief while complete healing was achieved by 8 or 12 weeks in 74–96% of the patients (compared with 28–66% for H_2 antagonists) (Figure 3.2). Omeprazole was effective whatever the severity of the oesophagitis. An improvement in symptoms is usually paralleled by healing [35].

Of patients resistant to H_2-receptor antagonists and subsequently treated by omeprazole, 90% have achieved complete healing by 12

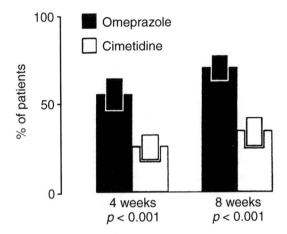

Figure 3.2 Healing of oesophagitis after 4 and 8 weeks of treatment with omeprazole (20 mg o.m.) or cimetidine (400 mg q.d.s.). (Source: redrawn from Bate CM, Keeling PWN, O'Morain C *et al.* Comparison of omeprazole and cimetidine in reflux oesophagitis: symptomatic, endoscopic and histological evaluations. *Gut* 1990; **31**: 968–972, with permission of the publisher.)

weeks (analysed by Sontag [15], based on seven studies including 478 patients).

Omeprazole 10 mg daily is less effective than 20 mg but more effective than ranitidine 150 mg b.d. [36].

Healing of the oesophagitis does not alter the underlying pathophysiology and if inadequate or no maintenance treatment is given more than 80% of healed patients have been shown to relapse within 6 months [35]. A meta-analysis of 1154 patients entered into five randomized maintenance trials have shown omeprazole 20 mg daily to maintain remission in approximately 80%, but in only 50% with 10 mg daily [37]. A higher relapse rate was associated with more severe pre-treatment oesophagitis and younger age.

Gastro-oesophageal reflux without oesophagitis

All of the above studies were confined to patients with oesophagitis as the changes are easy to measure endoscopically. However, at least 50% of patients with symptomatic reflux do not have oesophagitis. More recent randomized controlled trials have focused on this latter group. The first published study randomized 209 patients to receive either omeprazole 20 mg daily or a placebo for 4 weeks [38]. However, entry to the trial was on symptomatic assessment alone. Reflux was not confirmed by pH monitoring. The study might therefore have included a number of patients with 'functional heartburn'. A total of 57% of the patients in the study were rendered free of heartburn compared with only 19% receiving placebo. It may be of relevance that a favourable response to omeprazole was less likely in patients with symptoms of irritable bowel syndrome. In another trial with similar entry criteria, but in which oesophageal pH measurements were also performed, better responses to omeprazole were seen in the patients with the most abnormal oesophageal acid exposure [39].

Acid-sensitive oesophagus and functional heartburn

A double-blind crossover placebo-controlled trial of omeprazole 20 mg b.d. in patients with reflux symptoms but with normal endoscopy and normal total oesophageal acid exposure has now been carried out. Eleven out of 12 patients with a correlation between symptoms and acid reflux ('acid-sensitive oesophagus'), but only one out of six without a correlation ('functional heartburn') benefited from omeprazole [40].

The 'PPI-resistant' patient

Some patients will not be able to take omeprazole because of intolerance or allergy. In others conventional doses may result in a poor therapeutic reponse. A number of factors might contribute to resistance.

- **Inadequate dose and inappropriate timing.** Failure to respond to omeprazole is usually due to inadequate acid suppression, some patients requiring up to 160 mg daily [41–44]. This can readily be demonstrated by 24-hour combined oesophageal and gastric pH recording. Virtually all patients can be rendered sympton-free by appropriate dose manipulation [43,44]. Although omeprazole is usually given in the morning, it is more effective in some patients if given at night, or even twice or more times daily [44–46]. An alternative to increasing the dose of omeprazole, especially in the maintenance situation, is to add cisapride [26]. High doses of the other PPIs do not appear to have been evaluated in this situation.
- **'Volume reflux'.** Some patients with GOR characteristically regurgitate large volumes of fluid, often bile-stained, particularly at night. They frequently wake coughing and spluttering. As the acid suppression resulting from omeprazole should reduce the volume of gastric juice it seems probable the refluxate might have a duodenal origin. In one study in which duodenogastro-oesophageal reflux (DGOR) was assessed by HIDA scanning this concept was supported [47]. This needs to be repeated with the more easily analysable Bilitec technique for assessing DGOR (pp. 17–18). The frequency of this condition, if indeed

it is a separate entity, is unclear. As already pointed out the recently published series of 'omeprazole-resistant' patients reports control of reflux symptoms in virtually all patients if enough omeprazole is given [43,44].

● *Helicobacter* **infection.** Although *Helicobacter pylori* is of no direct relevance to the pathogenesis of gastro-oesophageal reflux it is now clear that the degree of acid suppression achievable by a given dose of omeprazole may be greater if the stomach is infected by *Helicobacter* [48]. Thus if *Helicobacter* is eradicated (see below) the dose requirements of omeprazole might increase.

● **Drugs.** The drugs that may impair sphincter function have been listed above (p. 26).

● **Psychological factors.** Although it is now appreciated that psychological factors may be important in GOR [14,49] their role in 'PPI-resistant' patients has not been explored. Certainly it is the author's experience that some patients with proven reflux disease resistant to omeprazole admit to stress as being a major factor in the symptoms and respond to appropriate therapy. Relaxation therapy has been shown to reduce reflux in some patients [14].

● **Wrong diagnosis.** Some patients with typical symptoms of GOR have no objective evidence for reflux (p. 2). They are usually referred to as having 'functional heartburn' and do not respond to omeprazole [40].

Long-term safety of proton-pump inhibitors, serum gastrin, ECL hyperplasia and *H. pylori*

There have long been concerns about the safety of continuous gastric acid suppression. However, with more than 10 years' clinical experience of omeprazole no serious problems have emerged.

Inevitably acid suppression will increase the serum gastrin concentration (a normal physiological response to hypochlorhydria), which in rodents may result in hyperplasia of the enterochromaffin-like (ECL) cells and carcinoid-like nodules [50]. These also occur in rats as a result of H_2-receptor antagonists [50,51]. Similar lesions may occur in the human in pernicious anaemia, but these lesions are entirely benign and do not produce carcinoid-type mediators [52]. Their only known clinical manifestation is occult bleeding and the lesions often regress spontaneously [53]. However, the serum gastrin concentrations in pernicious anaemia are much higher than in omeprazole-treated patients [52] and the nodules have not been described in the latter.

A potentially important effect of long-term PPI treatment relates to *H. pylori* infection. The latter can lead to atrophic gastritis/intenstinal metaplasa, which may eventually lead to carcinoma. In one study long-

term acid suppression, whether as a result of omeprazole, or surger]
vagotomy or antrectomy appeared to accelerate the process, at least a
as to atrophic gastritis/intestinal metaplasia [54]. Long-term omepra
had no such adverse effects on the non-infected gastric mucosa. Th
patients are being considered for long-term PPI therapy it might be
dent to check for *H. pylori* infection and eradicate if present. How(
another study has not been able to confirm that omeprazole accele:
these changes [55].

Other effects of long-term acid inhibition by PPIs include a theor(
risk of gut infection [56] and malabsorption [57], but these are r(
clinically relevant.

Lansoprazole/pantoprazole

The more recently available proton-pump inhibitors appear to be eq(
as effective as omeprazole in conventional doses [58,59] but limited
suggest that the absorption of lansoprazole (and to some extent
toprazole) may be hampered by food or antacids [60–62]. Unless t
some time before meals, which may be inconvenient for the pa(
bioavailability might therefore be unpredictable. This does not appe
be a problem with omeprazole [63]. However, there have been no (
comparisons between these compounds. For patients resistant to stan
doses only omeprazole has so far been shown to be effective when hi
doses are given (see above). Omeprazole may be more effecti\
preventing stricture recurrence (Chapter 5) and inducing regressi(
columnar-lined (Barrett's) oesophagus (Chapter 6).

Lansoprazole may interact with oral contraceptives [64].

NEWER AND ALTERNATIVE APPROACHES

As the most important defect in GOR is an increase in TLOSRs (pp. 1:
attempts have been made to reduce these pharmacologically. Mittal
[65], in healthy subjects, have found atropine may reduce the frequer
TLOSRs and associated reflux despite reducing basal sphincter pre:
Although of interest it is unclear whether anticholinergics may be eff(
clinically as they would also reduce gastric emptying [66].

Morphine has also been reported to reduce TLOSRs [67]. It v
therefore be of interest to evaluate the opioid kappa receptor a\
fedotizine, which appears to be safe in clinical practice [68].

TLOSRs in response to air distension of the stomach or fat ing(
may be at least partially mediated by cholecystokinin [69]. These

a fatty meal in patients with GOR may also be abolished by loxiglumide [71].

Other treatments that appear to be beneficial include nasal continuous positive airway pressure and chewing gum [72,73]. The latter works by increasing salivary flow, the role of which is discussed in Chapter 2.

PREGNANCY

Heartburn occurs in up to 50% of all pregnancies. It may come and go at any time, but is usually most troublesome during the last trimester. The symptoms rapidly resolve after parturition, but often recur in subsequent pregnancies. Investigations are not usually necessary. The mechanism for the reflux includes both reduced basal lower oesophageal sphincter pressures secondary to the hormonal changes and the effects of increased intra-abdominal pressure [74].

Antacids and H_2-receptor antagonists appear to be safe for the fetus [74]. There is much less data available for proton-pump inhibitors, but the manufacturers of omeprazole are aware of numerous uneventful pregnancies occurring with its use [75]. Chewing gum, to increase salivary flow [73], might be an alternative.

Reflux increases the risk of pulmonary aspiration during anaesthesia. This can largely be prevented by administering omeprazole 80 mg the night before elective caesarean section [76].

STRATEGY IN THE INDIVIDUAL PATIENT

At almost every level of management of uncomplicated GOR there remain unanswered questions. Unfortunately, therefore, a pragmatic approach is often necessary.

Initial presentation and investigation

If the patient presents over the age of 45 years with a short history of reflux symptoms it is generally agreed that endoscopy is mandatory as the symptoms might be the first manifestation of carcinoma. For the younger patient, particularly with symptoms of long duration, many would recommend blind treatment with the minimal effective therapy to control symptoms. This approach has the advantage of convenience to the patient and low cost. The disadvantage is that the physician will have no knowledge of whether there is mucosal damage or columnar-lined oesophagus, the symptoms being no guide to the degree of structural disease. Most recent reviewers agree that severe mucosal disease should be treated more aggressively [34,77]. Thus the findings of endoscopy might profoundly affect the choice of treatment.

Whether or not yet proven it seems likely, on the basis on the known beneficial effects of proton-pump inhibitors on healing of oesophagitis, preventing recurrence of stricture (Chapter 5) and at least partially regressing columnar-lined oesophagus (Chapter 6), that their long-term use will prevent progression of the disease if this is to occur (Chapter 1), and possibly even prevent carcinoma. The incidence of malignant transformation of columnar-lined oesophagus is approximately 1/100 patient years (Chapter 6). As it may be possible to control the columnar lining there would appear to be every reason to try to identify these patients.

A recent international review concluded that all patients should have at least one endoscopy in their lifetime [77]. The author strongly supports this view. However, in view of the prevalence of GOR the resource implications are substantial. Probably those with severe mucosal disease should subsequently undergo check endoscopy to confirm healing.

The main indication for oesophageal pH monitoring is to confirm the diagnosis in endoscopy-negative patients who fail to respond to a proton-pump inhibitor (Chapter 19).

Which treatment?

Once a diagnosis is made, either on the basis of symptoms or endoscopy, all patients should be advised of life-style modifications, particularly regarding their fat intake. If endoscopy has shown no or minimal oesophagitis it is reasonable to offer the patient minimally effective treatment as few of them will progress to more serious disease (Chapter 1). This can be done in a stepwise fashion commencing with antacids, with or without alginic acids. If these fail many would prescribe H_2-receptor antagonists, but omeprazole 10 mg daily is more effective and is not associated with tolerance. Some patients will need substantially higher doses of omeprazole. For maintenance treatment it is reasonable for the patient to adjust the dose as appropriate. Requirements in an individual vary from time to time, but the dose is rarely less than that necessary to control symptoms initially.

With more severe mucosal disease, whatever the patient's symptoms, proton-pump inhibitors are appropriate as these are the only drugs to heal the mucosa consistently (10–40 mg or more of omeprazole daily). Whether sufficient maintenance dose should be given to keep the patient in endoscopic remission or simply to control symptoms is uncertain.

If long-term proton-pump inhibitors are to be given it might be prudent to eradicate *Helicobacter* infection first, if this is present before commencing therapy but the evidence is contradictory (N.B.: testing for *Helicobacter* at endoscopy or by breath test in a patient being treated with omeprazole may lead to false-negative results).

If the patient is intolerant to a particular proton-pump inhibitor it is worth trying an alternative, but side-effects are usually similar with any of those currently available. Other treatments are substantially less effective, but combinations such as an H_2-receptor antagonist with cisapride can prove satisfactory [26]. Hopefully, developments with drugs to reduce TLOSRs will prove satisfactory in the foreseeable future. Chewing gum might be a helpful adjunct to therapy for some patients. In the author's experience intolerance to proton-pump inhibitors is the commonest reason for referring patients for anti-reflux surgery.

COST-EFFECTIVENESS OF OPTIONS FOR MEDICAL MANAGEMENT

Although substantially more effective than H_2-receptor antagonists in the management of gastro-oesophageal reflux, proton-pump inhibitors are more expensive. However, the cost-effectiveness of a drug is a much more complex issue, involving consideration of short- and long-term symptom relief, mucosal healing, possible prevention of complications and the effect on other health care costs including number of subsequent consultations and investigations. In addition one must consider non-medical costs to the patient such as the number of days lost from work.

Sridhar *et al.* [78] have reviewed published cost-effectiveness analyses of the options for medical management, none of which considers the non-medical costs to the patient. Inevitably such studies are open to criticism. Some are based merely on management of the first episode, while long-term analysis depends on assumed management algorithms. Despite these criticisms, all studies firmly conclude the cost-effective superiority of omeprazole over H_2-receptor antagonists, in terms of both initial and maintenance treatment.

Lansoprazole is marketed at a slightly lower price than omeprazole and there are claims for superior cost-effectiveness [79]. However, the adverse effect of meals on lansoprazole absorption must be borne in mind [60,61]. Although in the context of randomized controlled trials, in which patients have usually been instructed to take lansoprazole an hour before breakfast, it appears equally as effective as omeprazole, in the 'real world' many patients may find this difficult to achieve, which might lead to increased dose requirements.

REFERENCES

1. Nebel OT, Castell DO. Lower esophageal sphincter pressure changes after food ingestion. *Gastroenterology* 1972; **63**: 778–783.
2. Becker DJ, Sinclair J, Castell DO, Wu WC. A comparison of high and low fat meals on post-prandial esophageal acid exposure. *Am J*

Gastroenterol 1989; **84**: 782–786.

3. Mathus-Vliegen LMH, Tytgat GNJ. 24 hour pH measurements in morbid obesity: effects of massive overweight, weight loss and gastric distension. *Eur J Gastroenterol Hepatol* 1996; **8**: 635–640.

4. Kjellin A, Ramell S, Rössner S, Thor K. Gastroesophageal reflux in obese patients is not reduced by weight reduction. *Scand J Gastroenterol* 1996; **31**: 1047–1051.

5. Castell DO. Obesity and gastro-oesophageal reflux: is there a relationship? *Eur J Gastroenterol Hepatol* 1996; **8**: 625–626.

6. Wright LE, Castell DO. The adverse effect of chocolate on lower esophageal sphincter pressure. *Dig Dis* 1975; **20**: 703–707.

7. Vitale GC, Cheadle WG, Patel B *et al*. The effect of alcohol on nocturnal gastroesophageal reflux. *JAMA* 1987; **258**: 2077–2079.

8. Owendl B, Pfeiffer A, Pehl C *et al*. Effect of decaffeination of coffee or tea on gastro-oesophageal reflux. *Aliment Pharmacol Ther* 1994; **8**: 283–287.

9. Stanciu C, Bennett JR. Smoking and gastro-oesophageal reflux. *Br Med J* 1972; **3**: 793–795.

10. Kahrilas PJ, Gupta RR. Mechanism of acid reflux associated with cigarette smoking. *Gut* 1990; **31**: 4–10.

11. Johnson LF, DeMeester TR. Evaluation of the head of the bed, bethanechol, and antacid foam tablets on gastroesophageal reflux. *Dig Dis Sci* 1981; **26**: 673–680.

12. Harvey RF, Gordon PC, Hadley N *et al*. Effects of sleeping with the bed-head raised and of ranitidine in patients with severe peptic oesophagitis. *Lancet* 1987; **ii**: 1200–1203.

13. Gallup. *Gallup Survey of Heartburn Across America*. Princeton, NJ: Gallup Organization, 1988.

14. McDonald-Haile J, Bradley LA, Bailey MA *et al*. Relaxation training reduces symptoms and acid exposure in patients with gastroesophageal reflux disease. *Gastroenterology* 1994; **107**: 61–69.

15. Sontag SJ. Rolling review: gastro-oesophageal reflux disease. *Aliment Pharmacol Ther* 1993; **7**: 293–312.

16. Ramirez B, Richter JE. Review article: Promotility drugs in the treatment of gastro-oesophageal reflux disease. *Aliment Pharmacol Ther* 1993; **7**: 5–20.

17. Ceccatelli P, Janssens J, van Trappen G *et al*. Cisapride restored the decreased lower oesophageal sphincter pressure in reflux patients. *Gut* 1988; **29**: 631–635.

18. Patterson WG, Wang H, Beck IT. The effect of cisapride in patients with reflux esophagitis: an ambulatory esophageal manometry/pH-metry study. *Am J Gastroenterol* 1997; **92**: 226–230.

19. Goldin GF, Marcinkiewicz M, Zbroch T *et al*. Esophagoprotective potential of cisapride. An additional benefit for gastroesophageal

reflux disease. *Dig Dis Sci* 1997; **42**: 1362–1369.

20. Tytgat GNJ, Janssens J, Reynolds JC, Wienbeck M. Update on the pathophysiology and management of gastro-oesophageal reflux disease. The role of prokinetic therapy. *Eur J Gastroenterol Hepatol* 1996; **8**: 603–611.

21. Galmiche J-P, Brandstätter G, Evreux M *et al.* Combined therapy with cisapride and cimetidine in severe reflux oesophagitis: a double blind controlled trial. *Gut* 1988; **29**: 675–681.

22. Inauen W, Emde C, Weber B *et al.* Effects of ranitidine and cisapride on acid reflux and oesophageal motility in patients with reflux oesophagitis: a 24 hour ambulatory combined pH and manometry study. *Gut* 1993; **34**: 1025–1031.

23. Tytgat GNJ, Anker-Hansen OJ, Carling L *et al.* Effect of cisapride on relapse of reflux oesophagitis healed with an anti-secretory drug. *Scand J Gastroenterol* 1992; **27**: 175–183.

24. Toussaint J, Gossuin A, Deruyttere M *et al.* Healing and prevention of relapse of reflux oesophagitis by cisapride. *Gut* 1991; **32**: 1280–1285.

25. Blum AL, Adami B, Bouzo MH *et al.* Effect of cisapride on relapse of oesophagitis: a multi-national placebo-controlled trial in patients healed with an anti-secretory drug. *Dig Dis Sci* 1993; **38**: 551–560.

26. Vigneri S, Termini R, Leandro G *et al.* A comparison of five maintenance therapies for reflux esophagitis. *N Engl J Med* 1995; **333**: 1106–1110.

27. Tytgat GNJ, Blum AL, Verlinden M. Prognostic factors for relapse and maintenance treatment with cisapride in gastro-oesophageal reflux disease. *Aliment Pharmacol Ther* 1995; **9**: 271–280.

28. Bell NJV, Burget D, Howden CW *et al.* Appropriate acid suppression for the management of gastro-oesophageal reflux disease. *Digestion* 1992; **51**(Suppl 1): 59–67.

29. de Caestecker JS, Blackwell JN, Pryde A, Heading RC. Daytime gastro-oesophageal reflux is important in oesophagitis. *Gut* 1987; **28**: 519–526.

30. Merki HS, Halter F, Wilder-Smith C *et al.* Effect of food on H_2-receptor blockade in normal subjects and duodenal ulcer patients. *Gut* 1990; **31**: 148–150.

31. Nwokolo CU, Pruitt EJ, Sawyerr AFM *et al.* Tolerance during five months of dosing with ranitidine 150 mg nightly: a placebo-controlled, double-blind study. *Gastroenterology* 1991; **101**: 948–953.

32. Wilder-Smith CH, Merki HS. Tolerance during dosing with H_2-receptor antagonists. *Scand J Gastroenterol* 1992; **27**(Suppl 193): 14–19.

33. Hurlimann S, Abbühl B, Inauen W, Halter F. Comparison of acid inhibition by either oral high-dose ranitidine or omeprazole. *Aliment Pharmacol Ther* 1994; **8**: 193–201.

34. Bell NJV, Hunt RH. Role of gastric acid suppression in the treatment of gastro-oesophageal reflux disease. *Gut* 1992; **33**: 118–124.
35. Hetzel DJ, Dent J, Reed WD *et al*. Healing and relapses of severe peptic esophagitis after treatment with omeprazole. *Gastroenterology* 1988; **95**: 903–912.
36. Venables TL, Newland RD, Patel AC *et al*. Omeprazole 10 mg once daily, omeprazole 20 mg once daily, or ranitidine 150 mg twice daily, evaluated as initial therapy for the relief of symptoms of gastro-oesophageal reflux disease in general practice. *Scand J Gastroenterol* 1997; **32**: 965–973.
37. Carlsson R, Galmiche J-P, Dent J *et al*. Prognostic factors influencing relapses of oesophagitis during maintenance therapy with anti-secretory drugs: a meta-analysis of long-term omeprazole trials. *Aliment Pharmacol Ther* 1997; **ii**: 473–482.
38. Bate CM, Griffin SM, Keeling PWN *et al*. Reflux symptom relief with omeprazole in patients without unequivocal oesophagitis. *Aliment Pharmacol Ther* 1996; **10**: 547–555.
39. Lindt, Havelund T, Carlsson R *et al*. Heartburn without oesophagitis: efficacy of omeprazole therapy and features determining therapeutic response. *Scand J Gastroenterol* 1997; **32**: 974–979.
40. Watson RGP, Tham TCK, Johnston BT, McDougall NI. Double blind cross-over placebo-controlled study of omeprazole in the treatment of patients with reflux symptoms and physiological levels of acid reflux – the 'sensitive oesophagus'. *Gut* 1997; **40**: 587–590.
41. Klinkenberg-Knol EC, Meuwissen SGM. Combined gastric and oesophageal 24-hour pH monitoring and oesophageal manometry in patients with reflux disease, resistant to treatment with omeprazole. *Aliment Pharmacol Ther* 1990; **4**: 485–495.
42. Holloway RH, Dent J, Nrielvala F, Mackinnon AM. Relation between oesophageal acid exposure and healing of oesophagitis with omeprazole in patients with severe reflux oesophagitis. *Gut* 1996; **38**: 649–654.
43. Leite LP, Johnston BT, Just RJ, Castell DO. Persistent acid secretion during omeprazole therapy: a study of gastric acid profiles in patients demonstrating failure of omeprazole therapy. *Am J Gastroenterol* 1996; **91**: 1527–1531.
44. Hendel J, Hendel L, Hage E *et al*. Monitoring of omeprazole treatment in gastro-oesophageal reflux disease. *Eur J Gastroenterol Hepatol* 1996; **8**: 417–420.
45. Hendel J, Hendel L, Aggestrup S. Morning or evening dosage of omeprazole for gastro-oesophageal reflux disease? *Aliment Pharmacol Ther* 1995; **9**: 693–697.
46. Kuo B, Castell DO. Optimal dosing of omeprazole 40 mg daily: effect on gastric and esophageal pH and serum gastrin in healthy controls.

Am J Gastroenterol 1996; **91**: 1532–1538.

47. Lobo, AJ, Barlow A, Bhonsle U *et al.* 'Volume reflux' in patients with symptoms poorly responsive to omeprazole is associated with enterogastric reflux of bile. *Gut* 1993; **34**(Suppl 1): S17.

48. Verdú EF, Armstrong D, Fraser R *et al.* Effect of *Helicobacter pylori* status on intragastric pH during treatment with omeprazole. *Gut* 1995; **36**: 539–543.

49. Johnston BT, Lewis SA, Love AHG. Psychological factors in gastro-oesophageal reflux disease. *Gut* 1995; **36**: 481–482.

50. Betton GR, Dormer CS, Wells T *et al.* Gastric ECL cell hyperplasia and carcinoids in rodents following chronic administration of H_2-antagonists SK & F 93479 and oxmetidine and omeprazole. *Toxicol Pathol* 1988; **16**: 288–298.

51. Bilchik AJ, Nilsson O, Modlin IM *et al.* H_2-receptor blockade induces peptide yy and enteroglucagon-secreting gastric carcinoids in mastomys. *Surgery* 1989; **106**: 1119–1126.

52. Harvey RF, Bradshaw MJ, Davidson CM *et al.* Multifocal gastric carcinoid tumours, achlorhydria and hypergastrinaemia. *Lancet* 1985; i: 951–954.

53. Harvey RF. Spontaneous resolution of multifocal gastric enterochromaffin-like carcinoid tumours. *Lancet* 1988; i: 821.

54. Kuipers EJ, Lundell L, Klinkenberg-Knol EC *et al.* Atrophic gastritis and *Helicobacter pylori* infection in patients with reflux esophagitis treated with omeprazole or fundoplication. *N Engl J Med* 1996; **334**: 1018–1012.

55. Lundell L, Havu N, Andersson A *et al.* Gastritis development and acid suppression revisited. Results of a randomised clinical study with long-term follow up. *Gastroenterology* 1997; **112**: A771.

56. Larner AJ, Hamilton MIR. Review article: Infective complications of therapeutic gastric acid inhibition. *Aliment Pharmacol Ther* 1994; **8**: 579–584.

57. Koop H. Review article: Metabolic consequences of long-term inhibition of acid secretion by omeprazole. *Aliment Pharmacol Ther* 1992; **6**: 399–406.

58. Berstad A, Hatlebakk JG. Lansoprazole in the treatment of reflux oesophagitis: a survey of clinical studies. *Aliment Pharmacol Ther* 1993; 7(Suppl 1): 34–36.

59. Mössner J, Hölscher EH, Herz R, Schneider A. A double-blind study of pantoprazole and omeprazole in the treatment of reflux oesophagitis: a multicentre trial. *Aliment Pharmacol Ther* 1995; **9**: 321–326.

60. Delhotal-Landes B, Cournot A, Vermerie N *et al.* The effect of food and antacids on lansoprazole absorption and disposition. *Eur J Drug Metab Pharmacokinet* 1991 (Special Issue No.3); 315–320.

61. Bergstrand R, Grind M, Nyberg G, Olofsson B. Decreased oral bioavailability of lansoprazole in healthy volunteers when given a standardised breakfast. *Clin Drug Invest* 1995; **9**: 67–71.

62. Benet LZ, Zech LZ. Pharmacokinetics – a relevant factor for the choice of a drug? *Aliment Pharmacol Ther* 1994; **8**(Suppl 1): 25–32.

63. Andersson T, Andrën K, Cederberg C *et al*. Bioavailability of omeprazole as enteric coated (EC) granules in conjunction with food on the first and seventh days of treatment. *Drug Invest* 1990; **2**: 184–188.

64. Colin-Jones DG. Safety of lansoprazole. *Aliment Pharmacol Ther* 1993; **7**(Suppl I): 56–60.

65. Mittal RK, Chiareli C, Liu J *et al*. Atropine inhibits gastric distension and pharyngeal receptor mediated lower oesophageal sphincter relaxation. *Gut* 1997; **41**: 285–290.

66. Janssens J, Sifrim D. Spontaneous transient lower esophageal sphincter relaxation. A target for treatment of gastroesophageal reflux disease. *Gastroenterology* 1995; **109**: 1703–1706.

67. Penagini R, Bianchi PA. Effect of morphine on gastroesophageal reflux and transient lower esophageal sphincter relaxation. *Gastroenterology* 1997; **113**: 409–414.

68. Reid NW, Abitbol JL, Bardhan KD *et al*. Efficacy and safety of the peripheral kappa agonist fedotozine versus placebo in the treatment of functional dyspepsia. *Gut* 1997; **41**: 664–668.

69. Boulant J, Fioramonti J, Dapoigny M *et al*. Cholecystokinin and nitric oxide in transient lower esophageal sphincter relaxations due to gastric distension in dogs. *Gastroenterology* 1994; **107**: 1059–1066.

70. Boulant J, Mathieu S, D'Amato M *et al*. Cholecystokinin in transient lower oesophageal sphincter relaxation due to gastric distension in humans. *Gut* 1997; **40**: 575–581.

71. Trudgill N, D'Amato M, Riley S. Loxiglumide inhibits post-prandial transient lower oesophageal sphincter relaxations in patients with gastro-oesophageal reflux disease. *Gut* 1997; **40**(Suppl 1): A32.

72. Kerr P, Shoenut JP, Steens RD *et al*. Nasal continuous positive airway pressure. A new treatment for nocturnal gastroesophageal reflux? *J Clin Gastroenterol* 1993; **17**: 276–280.

73. Schönfeld J, Hector M, Evans DF, Wingate DL. Oesophageal acid and salivary secretion: is chewing gum a treatment option for gastro-oesophageal reflux? *Digestion* 1997; **58**: 111–114.

74. Baron TH, Richter JE. Gastroesophageal reflux disease in pregnancy. *Gastroenterol Clin North Am* 1992; **21**: 777–791.

75. Personal communication from Astra Pharmaceuticals.

76. Morre J, Flynn RJ, Sampaio M *et al*. Effect of single-dose omeprazole on intragastric acidity and volume during obstetric anaesthesia. *Anaesthesia* 1989; **44**: 559–562.

77. Freston JW, Malagelada JR, Petersen H, McCloy RF. Critical issues in the management of gastroesophageal reflux disease. *Eur J Gastroenterol Hepatol* 1995; **7**: 577–586.
78. Sridhar S, Huang J, O'Brien BJ, Hunt RH. Clinical economics review: cost-effectiveness of treatment alternatives for gastro-oesophageal reflux disease. *Aliment Pharmacol Ther* 1996; **10**: 865–873.
79. Hatlebakk JG, Berstad A, Carling L *et al.* Lansoprazole versus omeprazole in short-term treatment of reflux oesophagitis: results of a Scandinavian multicentre trial. *Scand J Gastroenterol* 1993; **28**: 224–228.

4

Gastro-oesophageal reflux – surgical treatment

Among physicians surgery for gastro-oesophageal reflux sometimes has a poor reputation, for which there may be several justifiable reasons. Surgery may be undertaken for inappropriate indications, in particular for repair of a radiologically demonstrated hiatus hernia rather than for reflux (these are not synonymous: p. 13–15) and for patients with a history suggestive of reflux but in whom there has been no objective evidence for the diagnosis. Results will inevitably be poor for each of these patient groups. The problem may be compounded by the fact that general surgeons may carry out the procedure only rarely.

It is sometimes difficult to give credibility to the apparently excellent results of large published series. A British surgeon, Cuschieri [1], points out that 'the generally held view among surgeons that the commonly used anti-reflux operations are successful in some 80% of patients is based on incompletely audited experience and remains unsubstantiated'. He goes on to say that the majority of published series are retrospective, with few prospective long-term studies and that surgery may not produce the desired result in as many as 40% of patients. It must also be remembered that even in the most experienced hands there is a mortality associated with any major operative procedure.

Despite these comments there is no doubt whatsoever that excellent results can be achieved by experienced surgeons performing operations on properly selected patients [2].

INDICATIONS FOR SURGERY

The indications for surgery are relative. It is reasonable to consider surgery if there has been a poor response to medical treatment, if it is the patient's preference, if complications exist that are not controlled adequately by conventional management, or sometimes for economic reasons.

Poor response to medical treatment

For patients who are intolerant of or allergic to proton-pump inhibitors surgery may be the only viable option (p. 28). However, resistance to omeprazole, if given in high doses and appropriately timed, is unusual (p. 30). Surgery is often carried out for 'volume reflux', characterized by regurgitation of large quantities of fluid rather than heartburn. High doses of omeprazole in this situation do not appear to have been critically evaluated (pp. 30–31).

Patient preference

Some patients may refuse to take medication on a long-term basis, even though it is effective. The surgical option is perfectly reasonable provided the risks of operation are fully explained to the patient.

Complications

Surgery may be indicated for recurrent stricture and possibly for columnar-lined (Barrett's) oesophagus and for respiratory complications of reflux. These are discussed more fully in Chapters 5–7.

Economic reasons

Proton-pump inhibitors are expensive. At current prices a 1-year supply of omeprazole 20 mg daily costs £362. However, prices inevitably fall when drugs lose their patent. A recent analysis from Holland calculated the cost of treating the average patient with continuous omeprazole for 4 years is equivalent to the cost of an open fundoplication [3]. The break-even point for a laparoscopic fundoplication was 1.4 years. An analysis from the USA assessed the costs of omeprazole and laparoscopic fundoplication to favour the latter only after 10 years [4].

PREOPERATIVE ASSESSMENT

Before surgery is seriously contemplated it is absolutely essential to confirm that the patient has gastro-oesophageal reflux. A typical history alone is not adequate. It is increasingly recognized that a group of patients with apparently typical symptoms do not have objective evidence of reflux. Apart from having a normal endoscopy they have normal 24-hour oesophageal acid exposure and no correlation between 'physiological' periods of acid reflux and symptoms, and they fail to respond to omeprazole [5]. In view of their failure to respond to medical treatment there is a temptation to proceed to surgery, but there is absolutely no reason to suppose that they will benefit. They probably represent a variant of irritable bowel syndrome (p. 2).

A typical history with unequivocal endoscopic oesophagitis is acceptable evidence for reflux, but 24-hour ambulatory oesophageal pH monitoring must be carried out to confirm reflux in patients with normal endoscopy or an atypical history.

The role of preoperative oesophageal manometry is less clear. In the past it has been considered mandatory so that the type of operation can be tailored to the patient's oesophageal peristaltic activity [6]. However, it has recently been shown that the outcome following either an open [7] or laparoscopic [8] loose fundoplication is not influenced by preoperative manometric findings.

Preoperative manometry is important to exclude achalasia and scleroderma, each of which may present with symptoms difficult to distinguish from straightforward gastro-oesophageal reflux (pp. 86 and 129). A standard anti-reflux operation is inappropriate for either of these conditions.

SURGICAL OPTIONS

The procedures to be discussed include fundoplication, Angelchik prosthesis and endoscopic techniques.

Fundoplication

A fundoplication incorporates and maintains part of the distal oesophagus into the stomach to ensure it will be affected by changes in intra-abdominal pressure. The crural defect of the diaphragm is usually repaired. The operation is preferably carried out through the abdomen as the transthoracic approach is often complicated by troublesome pain.

The Nissen 360° wrap has been the most widely used in the past [9]. However, if the wrap is too tight there is a high prevalence of unacceptable dysphagia and inability to belch ('gas bloat') or vomit. Various partial and other wraps have therefore been described to reduce the complications, perhaps the most widely used operation now being the 'floppy Nissen', a loose 360° wrap [10].

Fundoplication has been reported to reduce by 50% the rate of transient lower oesophageal sphincter relaxations, the commonest mechanism for abnormal reflux [11] (pp. 12–13). This may be because the fundus is no longer available for distension, one of the stimuli to TLOSRs. In the same study it was also found that the number of TLOSRs accompanied by reflux also fell substantially, from 47% to 17%, probably because of the creation of the high-pressure zone around the lower oesophageal sphincter by the fundoplication.

Most studies have failed to demonstrate an improvement in disordered oesophageal peristalsis following fundoplication [12,13], but in one study there was an improvement accompanied by improved swallowing [8].

Complications of fundoplication

Although, if carried out by an experienced surgeon for the correct indications following appropriate preoperative investigations, the results of fundoplication are usually highly satisfactory [2], complications are not uncommon. These include dysphagia, gas bloat/difficulty in vomiting, and relapse of reflux.

Wo *et al.* [14] have recently reviewed the world literature relating to post-fundoplication dysphagia. Transient dysphagia has been reported in up to 70% of patients, but usually resolves spontaneously within 3 months. Persistent dysphagia has been reported in up to 24%. Often this is due to faulty surgical technique. In their own series of 35 patients with persisting dysphagia, a specific cause was found in 18, including a slipped fundoplication in 14 (identified by radiology and/or endoscopy), an oesophageal motility disorder in five and a stricture in four, more than one cause being found in some patients. For those with stricture or no apparent cause simple bougie dilatation was successful in relieving the symptoms in 12 of 18 patients, but in only three of 11 with a slipped fundoplication. For the patients in whom dilatation failed surgical revision was usually necessary.

Gas bloat and difficulty in vomiting are extremely unpleasant symptoms and are usually due to the wrap being too tightly applied to the oesophagus. They are much less common after a loose wrap [10].

Although fundoplication usually controls reflux well in the short term late failures are now well documented, with a reported prevalence of up to 26% at 10 years [15,16].

Laparoscopic fundoplication

In recent years there has been an explosion of interest in and enthusiasm for laparoscopic fundoplication. Short-term results are good and comparable to open surgery [17,18], but randomized controlled trials with long-term follow-up will be necessary to establish whether there are important differences in outcome between the two procedures.

Angelchik prosthesis

This is a silicone 'doughnut'-looking device that is tied around the bottom of the oesophagus [19]. It has the benefit of being a relatively simple operation to perform and in one series was as effective as an open fundoplication [20]. However, in another series seven out of 30 patients randomized to an Angelchik prosthesis had persisting severe oesophagitis, compared with none out of 31 in the fundoplication group [21]. Side-effects include gas bloat, dysphagia in 30–50%, migration of prosthesis, erosion into the alimentary tract, slippage or rotation with alimentary obstruction, and sepsis [21–24]. Because of these complications the procedure is now rarely carried out.

Endoscopic techniques

Swain and colleagues have devised an endoscopic method of achieving gastroplasty, fundoplication and anterior gastropexy [25]. In beagle dogs they have found the gastroplasty to be the most promising, achieved by suturing the anterior and posterior wall of the stomach to create a gastric tube (neo-oesophagus) along the lesser curve. Preliminary results in 28 patients have been reported [26]. The procedure was carried out as a day-case under benzodiazepine sedation. Good control of reflux was reported. The procedure has the advantage of easy repeatability.

REFERENCES

1. Cuschieri A. Surgical treatment of reflux disease. In: Hennessy TPJ, Cuschieri A, Bennett JR, eds. *Reflux Oesophagitis*. London: Butterworths, 1989: pp 143–169.
2. Spechler SJ. Comparison of medical and surgical therapy for complicated gastroesophageal reflux disease in veterans. *N Engl J Med* 1992; **326:** 786–792.
3. Van den Boom G, Go PMMYH, Hameeteman W *et al*. Cost effectiveness of medical versus surgical treatment in patients with severe or refractory gastroesophageal reflux disease in the Netherlands. *Scand J Gastroenterol* 1996; **31:** 1–9.
4. Heudebert GR, Marks R, Wilcox CM, Centor RM. Choice of long-term strategy for the management of patients with severe esophagitis: a cost-utility analysis. *Gastroenterology* 1997; **112:** 1078–1086.
5. Watson RGP, Tham TCK, Johnston BT, McDougall NI. Double blind cross-over placebo controlled study of omeprazole in the treatment of patients with reflux symptoms and physiological levels of acid reflux – the 'sensitive oesophagus'. *Gut* 1997; **40:** 587–590.
6. DeMeester TR, Peters JH. Surgical treatment of gastroesophageal reflux disease. In: Castell DO, ed. *The Esophagus*. 2nd ed. Boston, MA: Little, Brown, 1995: pp 577–617.
7. Mughal MM, Bancewicz J, Marples M. Oesophageal manometry and pH recording does not predict the bad results of Nissen fundoplica-

tion. *Br J Surg* 1990; **77**: 43–45.

8. Baigrie RJ, Watson DI, Myers JC, Jamieson GG. Outcome of laparoscopic Nissen fundoplication in patients with disordered preoperative peristalsis. *Gut* 1997; **40**: 381–185.

9. Nissen R. Eine einfache Operation zur Beeinflussung der Refluxösophagitis. *Schweiz Med Wschr* 1956; **86**: 590–592.

10. Donahue PE, Samelson S, Nyhus LM, Bombeck CT. The floppy Nissen fundoplication. Effective long-term control of pathological reflux. *Arch Surg* 1985; **120**: 663–668.

11. Ireland AC, Holloway RH, Toouli J, Dent J. Mechanisms underlying the anti-reflux action of fundoplication. *Gut* 1993; **34**: 303–308.

12. Russel COH, Pope CHE, Gannan RM *et al.* Does surgery correct esophageal motor dysfunction in gastroesophageal reflux? *Am Surgeon* 1981; **194**: 290–296.

13. Behar J, Sheahan DG, Biancani P *et al.* Medical and surgical management of reflux esophagitis, a 38 month report on a prospective clinical trial. *N Engl J Med* 1975; **293**: 263–268.

14. Wo JM, Trus TL, Richardson WS *et al.* Evaluation and management of postfundoplication dysphagia. *Am J Gastroenterol* 1996; **91**: 2318–2322.

15. Siewert JR, Feussner H. Early and long-term results of anti-reflux surgery: a critical look. *Clin Gastroenterol* 1987; **1**: 821–842.

16. Negre JB, Markkulh HT, Keyrilainen O *et al.* Nissen fundoplication. Results at 10 year follow up. *Am J Surg* 1983; **146**: 635–638.

17. Peters JH, Heimbucher J, Kauer WKH *et al.* Clinical and physiological comparison of laparoscopic and open Nissen fundoplication. *J Am Coll Surg* 1995; **180**: 385–393.

18. Alderson D, Welbourn CRB. Laparoscopic surgery for gastro-oesophageal reflux disease. *Gut* 1997; **40**: 565–567.

19. Angelchik JP, Cohen RA. A new surgical procedure for the treatment of gastroesophageal reflux and hiatal hernia. *Surg Gynecol Obstet* 1979; **148**: 246–248.

20. Gear MWL, Gilleson EW, Dowling BL. Randomised prospective trial of the Angelchik anti-reflux prosthesis. *Br J Surg* 1984; **71**: 681–683.

21. Stewart RC, Dawson K, Keeling P *et al.* A prospective randomised trial of Angelchik prosthesis versus Nissen fundoplication. *Br J Surg* 1989; **76**: 86–89.

22. Wale RJ, Royston CMS, Bennett JR, Buckton GK. Prospective study of the Angelchik anti-reflux prosthesis. *Br J Surg* 1985; **72**: 520–524.

23. Pickleman J. Disruption and migration of an Angelchik esophageal anti-reflux prosthesis. *Surgery* 1983; **93**: 467–468.

24. Lilly MP, Slapsky SF, Thompson WR. Intraluminal erosion and migration of the Angelchik anti-reflux prosthesis. *Arch Surg* 1984; **119**: 849–853.

25. Kadirkamanathan SS, Evans DF, Gong F *et al.* Anti-reflux operations at flexible endoscopy using endoluminal stitching techniques: an experimental study. *Gastrointest Endosc* 1996; **44**: 133–143.
26. Swain CP, Kadirkamanathan SS, Gong F, Evans D. Endoscopic gastroplasty for gastro-oesophageal reflux disease. *Gut* 1997; **40**(Suppl 1): A34.

5

Gastro-oesophageal reflux – ulcers and stricture

Although ulcers and stricture are often secondary to gastro-oesophageal reflux there are other causes (Table 5.1). These include malignancy (Chapter 12), drugs (Chapter 16), corrosives (Chapter 16), infections (Chapter 11), cutaneous diseases (Chapter 13), after variceal sclerotherapy, post-radiation, connective tissue diseases and Crohn's disease (Chapter 16). Biopsy and other investigations will often be necessary to clarify the diagnosis. Additional causes for stricture include after

Table 5.1 Causes of oesophageal ulcers and stricture

- Causes of ulcers and stricture
  - Gastro-oesophageal reflux
  - Malignancy
  - Drugs
  - Corrosives
  - Infections
  - Cutaneous diseases
  - Post-variceal sclerotherapy
  - Radiation
  - Connective tissue diseases
  - Crohn's disease
- Additional causes of stricture
  - Post-fundoplication
  - Post-surgical resection
  - Webs/rings

---

surgery (fundoplication, oesophageal or oesophageal/gastric resection) and webs/rings (Chapter 14).

ULCERS IN GASTRO-OESOPHAGEAL REFLUX

Acid–peptic erosions and ulcers differ only in severity. Erosions are defined as lesions confined to the mucosa whereas ulcers penetrate the muscularis mucosa. They may also complicate columnar-lined (Barrett's) oesophagus (Chapter 6). Ulcers are more likely to be associated with severe bleeding than erosions and may perforate into the mediastinum, pleura or aorta. Perforations are thus a potentially serious complication.

Usually, reflux-induced ulcers heal with acid suppression [1], but if not the other causes for ulcers listed in Table 5.1 should be considered.

STRICTURE IN GASTRO-OESOPHAGEAL REFLUX

Gastro-oesophageal reflux is by far the commonest cause of a benign oesophageal stricture, accounting for 214 of 254 patients in one series [2].

A reflux-induced stricture occurs primarily in the distal oesophagus. It is often only a few millimetres in length, but may be much more extensive and involve almost the whole oesophagus. In one series columnar-lined oesophagus was present in 44% [3], in which cases the stricture may occur more proximally.

Drug ingestion, particularly NSAIDs, have been implicated in the pathogenesis of a substantial number of strictures related to reflux disease [4,5].

Most patients give a long history of symptoms of reflux, but these may be absent, dysphagia being the first presentation in 25% of patients in one series [6]. Interestingly, patients with stricture are often edentulous [7]. This might be because the edentulous state results in less ingestion of solid food with less oesophageal dilatation and salivation to neutralize acid reflux. Alternatively, years of uncontrolled acid reflux may damage teeth [8].

Gradual onset of dysphagia is the cardinal manifestation of a stricture, but it is important to appreciate that dysphagia in a patient with known gastro-oesophageal reflux is just as likely to be due to severe oesophagitis [9] and may also be due to poor oesophageal motility [10].

If a stricture is suspected it is best first evaluated radiologically. Characteristically it is smooth and tapering (Figure 5.1).

A lumen of less than 12 mm diameter will cause dysphagia [11]. Endoscopically a discrete tight fibrous ring can usually be recognized (Plate 3), often with erosive oesophagitis or columnar metaplasia.

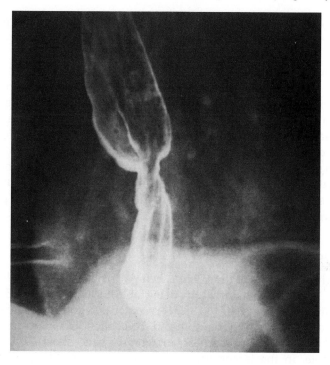

Figure 5.1 Barium swallow to illustrate the smooth nature of a benign oesophageal stricture.

Cytology and biopsies should always be carried out to exclude malignancy and other unsuspected diagnoses (Table 5.1).

Treatment of acid–peptic stricture

The majority of strictures can be treated endoscopically under benzodiazepine sedation [2]. A guide wire is passed down the biopsy channel and through the stricture, under radiological control if necessary. The endoscope is then removed and a dilator is passed firmly over the guide wire. Two types of dilator are commonly used: increasing-sized metal olives (e.g. Eder–Puestow), or tapered rubber or plastic dilators, also of increasing sizes (e.g. Celestin or Savary–Gillard). It is important not to force the dilator and, with experience, to advance the instrument by 'feel'. Balloon dilators (e.g. Rigiflex) are now available. No guide wire is required, the balloon being passed down the biopsy channel and through the stricture. It can then be inflated under direct vision. A randomized controlled trial comparing olives with the balloon showed the former to be marginally more effective [12]. Dilatation to at least 12 mm should be aimed for, but preferably to 18 mm [2]. For very tight strictures it is prudent to achieve full dilatation in two or more sessions, 2–3 weeks apart.

The overall perforation rate of forceful dilatation of an oesophageal stricture is about 1% [2]. This can usually be recognized by chest/epigastric pain, dyspnoea, fever, tachycardia and surgical emphysema in the neck. Chest and neck X-rays may reveal air in the mediastinum and soft tissues but, if they are negative and a perforation is suspected, a radiographic contrast swallow using a water-soluble medium should be carried out. Small perforations can usually be treated conservatively, i.e. nil by mouth, gastric aspiration and antibiotics. Surgery should not be delayed where there is concern that the patient is not improving.

Prevention of recurrence

Although bougie dilatation of a benign stricture is usually highly effective, with the patient again being able to eat normally, 50% need re-dilatation within 1 year [6,13]. H_2-receptor antagonists do not prevent recurrence [14,15]. Two randomized controlled trials of omeprazole 20 mg daily against H_2-receptor antagonists have shown a benefit for omeprazole. In the larger study of Smith *et al.* [16] 366 patients were randomized after effective dilatation. At the end of 1 year of follow-up 43/143 of the omeprazole group, compared with 66/143 in the ranitidine group, needed re-dilatation. Similarly the average number of dilatations per patient was 0.48 with omeprazole and 1.08 with ranitidine. Both of these differences were statistically significant. Similar results have been found in a smaller trial [17].

A report of omeprazole 40 mg daily suggests much more effective prevention of recurrence. In a randomized study stricture recurrence was prevented in nine of 10 patients [18]. Furthermore, in the same study omeprazole appeared to be much more effective than either lansoprazole 60 mg daily or pantoprazole 80 mg daily, which only maintained remission in 20% and 30% of patients respectively.

Surgery for stricture

Fortunately, benign acid–peptic strictures rarely need resection. This is often an unsatisfactory operation with a high stricture recurrence rate [19].

For patients with rapidly recurrent 'dilatable' strictures a standard anti-reflux operation reduces or abolishes the need to re-dilate [20,21]. If an anti-reflux operation is difficult or not feasible a Roux-en-Y diversion has proved to be effective [22,23].

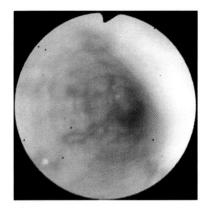

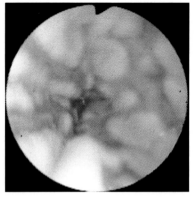

Plate 1 Non-confluent erosive oesophagitis (Savary–Miller stage I).

Plate 2 Circumferential erosive oesophagitis (Savary–Miller stage III).

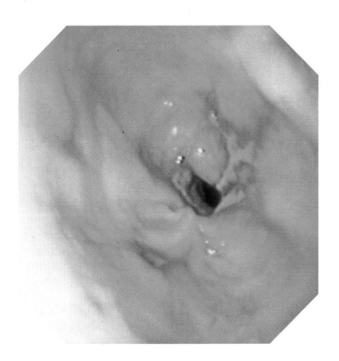

Plate 3 Endoscopic view of a benign oesophageal stricture, showing tight fibrous stricture above which there is erosive oesophagitis.

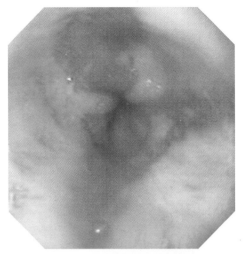

Plate 4 Endoscopic view of an irregular upper margin of columnar-lined oesophagus. Such 'fingers' of mucosa extending into the oesophagus may represent normal gastric mucosa. Biopsy is therefore essential to clarify their significance.

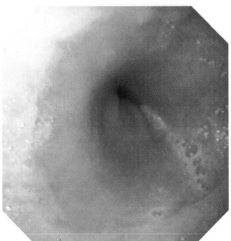

Plate 5 Endoscopic view of a regular upper margin of columnar-lined oesophagus.

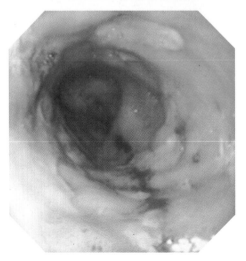

Plate 6 Multiple ulcers within columnar-lined oesophagus.

REFERENCES

1. Hetzel DJ, Dent J, Reed WD *et al*. Healing and relapse of severe peptic esophagitis after treatment with omeprazole. *Gastroenterology* 1988; **95**: 903–912.

2. Cox JGC, Bennett JR. Benign oesophageal strictures. In: Bennett JR, Hunt RH, eds. *Therapeutic Endoscopy and Radiology of the Gut*. 2nd ed. London: Chapman & Hall, 1990: pp 11–42.

3. Spechler SJ, Sterber H, Doos WG, Schimmel EM. The prevalence of Barrett's esophagus in patients with chronic peptic esophageal stricture. *Dig Dis Sci* 1983; **28**: 769–774.

4. Heller SR, Fellowes IW, Ogilvie AL, Atkinson M. Non-steroidal anti-inflammatory drugs and benign oesophageal stricture. *Br Med J* 1982; **285**: 167–168.

5. El-Serag HB, Sonnenberg A. Association of esophagitis and esophageal strictures with diseases treated with non-steroidal anti-inflammatory drugs. *Am J Gastroenterol* 1997; **92**: 52–56.

6. Patterson DJ, Graham DY, Lacey-Smith J *et al*. Natural history of benign esophageal stricture treated by dilatation. *Gastroenterology* 1983; **85**: 346–350.

7. Maxton DG, Ainley CC, Grainger SL *et al*. Teeth and benign oesophageal stricture. *Gut* 1987; **28**: 61–63.

8. Schroeder PL, Filler SJ, Ramirez B *et al*. Dental erosion and acid reflux disease. *Ann Intern Med* 1995; **12**: 809–815.

9. Dakkak M, Hoare RC, Maslin SC and Bennett JR. Oesophagitis is as important as oesophageal stricture diameter in determining dysphagia. *Gut* 1993; **34**: 152–155.

10. Singh S, Stein HJ, De Meester T, Hinder RA. Nonobstructive dysphagia in gastroesophageal reflux disease: a study with combined ambulatory pH and motility monitoring. *Am J Gastroenterol* 1992; **87**: 562–567.

11. Hennessy TPJ, Cuschieri A, Bennett JR. Benign strictures and other complications of reflux. In: Hennessy TPJ, Cuschieri A, Bennett JR, eds. *Reflux Oesophagitis*. London: Butterworths, 1989: pp 171–191.

12. Cox JGC, Winter RK, Maslin SC *et al*. Balloon or bougie for dilatation of benign oesophageal stricture? An interim report of a randomised controlled trial. *Gut* 1988; **29**: 1741–1747.

13. Hands IJ, Papavramidis S, Bishop H *et al*. The natural history of peptic oesophageal strictures treated by dilatation and anti-reflux therapy alone. *Ann R Coll Surg Engl* 1989; **71**: 306–309.

14. Ferguson R, Dronfield MW, Atkinson M. Cimetidine in treatment of reflux oesophagitis with peptic stricture. *Br Med J* 1979; **ii**: 472–474.

15. Farup PG, Modalsli B, Tholfsen JK. Long-term treatment with 300 mg ranitidine once daily after dilatation of peptic oesophageal strictures.

Scand J Gastroenterol 1992; **27**: 594–598.

16. Smith PM, Kerr GD, Cockel R *et al.* A comparison of omeprazole and ranitidine in the prevention of recurrence of benign esophageal stricture. *Gastroenterology* 1994; **107**: 1312–1318.

17. Marks RD, Richter JE, Rizzo J *et al.* Omeprazole versus H$_2$-receptor antagonists in treating patients with peptic stricture and esophagitis. *Gastroenterology* 1994; **106**: 907–915.

18. Jaspersen D, Diehl K-L, Schoeppner H *et al.* A comparison of omeprazole, lansoprazole and pantoprazole in the maintenance treatment of severe reflux oesophagitis. *Aliment Pharmacol Ther* 1998; **12**: 49–52.

19. Belsey RHR. Reconstruction of the esophagus with left colon. *J Thorac Cardiovasc Surg* 1965; **49**: 33–35.

20. Naef AP and Savary M. Conservative operations for peptic esophagitis with stenosis with columnar-lined lower esophagus. *Ann Thorac Surg* 1972; **13**: 543–551.

21. Watson A. The role of anti-reflux surgery combined with fibre-optic endoscopic dilatation in peptic esophageal stricture. *Am J Surg* 1984; **148**: 346–349.

22. Royston CMS, Dowling BL and Spencer J. Antrectomy with Roux-en-Y anastomosis in the treatment of peptic oesophagitis with stricture. *Br J Surg* 1975; **62**: 605–607.

23. Washer JF, Gear MWL, Dowling BL *et al.* Randomised prospective trial of Roux-en-Y duodenal diversion versus fundoplication for severe reflux oesophagitis. *Br J Surg* 1984; **71**: 181–184.

6

Gastro-oesophageal reflux – columnar-lined (Barrett's) oesophagus

What Barrett described in 1950 [1] is somewhat removed from what is now referred to as 'Barrett's oesophagus'. He identified peptic ulceration in columnar epithelium above a hiatus hernia, concluding that the ulcer was in part of the stomach located intrathoracically as a result of a congenitally short oesophagus. This had previously been described some 50 years earlier [2]. Allison and Johnstone [3] pointed out that the columnar epithelium was in fact lining the oesophagus, views subsequently accepted by Barrett, who suggested the term 'lower oesophagus lined by columnar epithelium' [4]. Moersch *et al.* [5] recognized the association with gastro-oesophageal reflux.

The importance of columnar-lined (Barrett's) oesophagus (CLO) lies in its relationship to the development of adenocarcinoma of the oesophagus and of the gastric cardia.

DEFINITION OF CLO

Traditionally, CLO is defined as a metaplastic columnar lining of the lower oesophageal tube of at least 3 cm in length, as this is easily defined endoscopically. If it is shorter than 3 cm it may be difficult or impossible to distinguish from normal gastric mucosa, which may line the lower 2 cm of the oesophagus [6].

Three types of histological change are recognized [7]. Adjacent to the normal gastric mucosa it may resemble the mucosa of the fundus, although the glands are sparse and short. Above this it may resemble the junctional gastric mucosa, but chief, parietal, Paneth and goblet cells are absent. Adjacent to the squamous epithelium of the oesophagus the usual type is incomplete intestinal metaplasia, also referred to as specialized intestinal metaplasia. Villi and goblet cells are present, but a well defined brush border is usually lacking. The goblet cell is the most important cell type for the diagnosis of intestinal metaplasia. Some otherwise normal cells of the gastric cardia can resemble goblet cells on simple H&E staining and do not indicate the presence of intestinal metaplasia. Staining with H&E–Alcian blue at pH 2.5 is therefore recommended to identify goblet cells unequivocally and so avoid overdiagnosis of CLO [8]. Intestinal metaplasia is the most prevalent histological type of abnormal mucosa and the one most often associated with development of carcinoma [9].

Clearly, histological confirmation of the diagnosis of CLO is always needed and there is an increasing tendency now to define the condition as present if there is histologically proven intestinal metaplasia anywhere in the lower oesophageal tube, regardless of extent [10].

Short-segment columnar-lined oesophagus

Although 3 cm of CLO is usually easy to recognize endoscopically, metaplastic columnar epithelium of shorter extent is relatively common with gastro-oesophageal reflux and must have biopsy confirmation of its presence for the reasons stated above. It may also predispose to adenocarcinoma [11,12].

Intestinal metaplasia may also be found in the columnar mucosa at a normally positioned squamocolumnar junction, i.e. within the mucosa of the gastric cardia. This has caused confusion about the meaning of 'short-segment columnar-lined (Barrett's) oesophagus'. Spechler *et al.* [13] took biopsies from the squamocolumnar junction of 142 unselected patients, i.e. with and without reflux symptoms, attending for routine diagnostic endoscopy. Those with more than 3 cm of CLO were excluded. No fewer than 26 (18%) had intestinal metaplasia within the columnar epithelium. In some the appearance of the squamocolumnar junction was that of 'fingers' extending into the lower oesophagus, but in others it was straight and coincided with the normally located oesophagogastric junction. Five other groups have similarly investigated unselected patients and found intestinal metaplasia with a prevalence of 8–36% (Table 6.1) [14–18].

Do these findings have the same significance as intestinal metaplasia in traditional long-segment columnar oesophagus, i.e. an association with reflux and predisposition to adenocarcinoma? In three of the six studies there was no detectable relationship with symptoms and/or endoscopic manifestations of reflux [13,16,18]. In one there was a definite relationship [14]. In another a relationship was claimed in the text, but not borne out by the data in the table [15]. In the final study, which may help to clarify the situation, the patients with intestinal metaplasia could be subdivided into those in whom it extended into the lower oesophagus and those with

Table 6.1 Findings relating to junctional intestinal metaplasia in unselected patients attending for diagnostic endoscopy

	Spechler et al. [13]	Johnston et al. [14]	Weston et al. [15]	Nandurkar et al. [16]	Chalasani et al. [17]	Trudgill et al. [18]
No. patients	142	170	239	158	87	120
Prevalence of intestinal metaplasia (%)	18	9	8	36	18	18
Reflux-related	No	Yes	?	No	Yes in subgroup	No
Age-related	Yes*	Yes*	Yes	Yes*	No	Yes

*Not statistically significant

intestinal metaplasia associated with a normally located squamocolumnar junction at the oesophagogastric junction. There was a relationship to reflux symptoms in only the former group, who probably therefore represent true short-segment columnar-lined (Barrett's) oesophagus. In the others in whom it is not secondary to reflux it might be a manifestation of intestinal metaplasia elsewhere in the stomach, a statistically significant relationship being found in the study of Trudgill *et al.* [18]. It is suggested that the term short-segment CLO be reserved for those patients in whom the instestinal metaplasia is within the oesophagus and related to reflux. Unfortunately, it may be difficult at endoscopy to define precisely the oesophagogastric junction and therfore the origin of the biopsies.

The intestinal metaplasia cannot be reliably recognized endoscopically. Its presence was confirmed histologically in only 19 of 40 suspected cases in the study of Weston *et al.* [15].

It is already established that true short-segment columnar-lined oesophagus has malignant potential (see above), but whether the other cases in whom there is no apparent relationship to reflux have a similar risk is unknown.

EPIDEMIOLOGY AND NATURAL HISTORY

Approximately 10% of patients with oesophagitis attending for endoscopy have underlying CLO [19]. It is progressively more prevalent with age, with a peak age of diagnosis in life after 60 years [20]. It is twice as common in males and more common in whites than blacks. Several reports point to an association with both smoking and alcohol consumption, but others have failed to confirm these [19]. It may have a familial tendency [21]. As would be anticipated it is frequently found in association with scleroderma oesophagus and treated achalasia, both conditions associated with gastro-oesophageal reflux. On the basis of cases diagnosed endoscopically and from unselected autopsies Cameron *et al.* [20] have estimated a true prevalence of 400/100 000 population, with only about 1/20 being diagnosed in life.

Limited prospective data suggests that CLO, at least in most patients, develops very rapidly after the onset of gastro-oesophageal reflux to reach its maximum length in 1–2 years [22]. The mean length of CLO is similar in any age group (Figure 6.1) [20]. Thus, although the prevalence increases with age, the length does not. This also supports the concept that CLO attains its full length early in its natural history and changes little thereafter, a concept supported by findings of long-term surveillance studies unless the patient develops dysplasia [23].

Progression to carcinoma is discussed below.

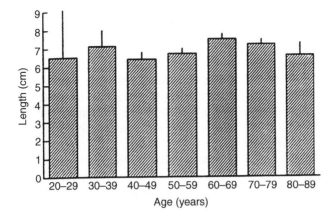

Figure 6.1 Mean length of columnar-lined (Barrett's) oesophagus in relation to age. Despite the increasing prevalence of CLO with age the length does not appear to change, suggesting that the abnormality reaches its full length early in its natural history. (Source: redrawn from reference 20, with permission of the publisher.)

SYMPTOMS

Unless accompanied by carcinoma, ulcer or stricture, CLO does not cause specific symptoms other than those of gastro-oesophageal reflux. Ulcer and stricture have been discussed in Chapter 5. Some patients give no history of symptoms of reflux [24] and as a group they appear to have a reduced oesophageal pain threshold to acid [25]. Whether the latter is a result of the abnormal epithelium being less sensitive or otherwise is unclear.

ENDOSCOPIC DIAGNOSIS OF CLO

Contrast radiology is unreliable in the diagnosis of CLO [26]. Diagnosis is dependent upon histology. Endoscopy is therefore essential.

Erosive oesophagitis may or may not be present. Otherwise it is usually easily recognized as velvety, dark salmon-pink mucosa extending more than 3 cm into the oesophagus from the proximal margin of the gastric folds. Its distal margins merge imperceptibly into the gastric mucosa. Proximally it contrasts sharply with the whitish, normal oesophageal squamous epithelium. The upper margin may be irregular and flame-like or circumferential (Plates 4, 5). Small columnar islands may be seen in the lower part of the squamous epithelium, or squamous islands within the upper part of the CLO. The latter are more often seen after treatment with proton-pump inhibitors [27] or anti-reflux surgery

[28]. Ulcers, which are often multiple (Plate 6), and strictures may be present within the CLO.

CLO may be more difficult to diagnose in patients with associated erosive oesophagitis. Even without oesophagitis the squamocolumnar junction is occasionally difficult to define [29]. The macroscopic appearance of possible CLO of less than 3 cm in length is unreliable. Fingers of columnar mucosa extending into the lower 1–2 cm of the oesophagus, a frequent endoscopic finding, do not necessarily indicate intestinal metaplasia (see above) [15].

Many patients with CLO have a sliding hiatus hernia.

The endoscopic appearance of CLO can be enhanced by dye spraying. Lugol's iodine (5 ml of 50% solution) stains the squamous epithelium black and may thus more clearly define the squamocolumnar junction [30]. Methylene blue will be taken up by intestinal metaplasia [31]. It also stains ulcers.

Intestinal metaplasia can also be clearly defined by magnification endoscopy, particularly after staining with 0.1% indigocarmine, while dysplastic areas may look raised [32].

High-grade dysplasia can be detected by laser-induced fluorescence spectroscopy. This is a use of light to discriminate different types of tissue *in situ*. Panjehpour *et al.* [33], using 410 nm light from a dye laser, were able to detect high-grade dysplasia with a specificity and sensitivity of more than 90%.

Brush cytology should be used in addition to pinch biopsies if malignancy is suspected [34].

Endoscopic ultrasound has been used to detect high-grade dysplasia and early carcinoma, but with variable results [35].

PATHOPHYSIOLOGY AND PATHOGENESIS

Jankowski [36] has suggested a mechanism for the development of CLO as an adaptive response to refluxed gastric and duodenal juice. Secondary to reflux damage to the squamous epithelium there is an increase in the height and length of the proliferative zone, resulting in a folding of the proliferative layer with papilla formation. Because of both damage to the surface epithelium and increased height of the papillae, the stem cells within the proliferative layer will now be more exposed to refluxate. This might promote the development of acid-resistant lineages (gastric metaplasia) and lineages resistant to the effects of duodenal juice (intestinal metaplasia).

The reason why some patients with gastro-oesophageal reflux develop CLO while others do not has not been resolved. A simplistic answer would be that those with CLO are the most severe refluxers, which would result in the greatest damage to the oesophageal squamous epithelium and therefore the greatest risk of exposure of stem cells to refluxate. This is supported by reports of patients with CLO, when compared with those with just oesophagitis, having lower values for basal lower oesophageal sphincter pressure [37], reduced oesophageal peristaltic amplitude [38] and more prolonged acid exposure and less effective acid clearance [37,39].

However, Neumann and Cooper [40] have pointed out that many of these earlier reports were from surgical units and might therefore have a bias towards patients with more complications. They also point out that the control subjects were either not age-matched or the ages were not given. This may be important since their own study has shown acid reflux is age-dependent. Using appropriate age-matched controls they could not confirm a difference in 24-hour oesophageal acid exposure between patients with severe oesophagitis alone and those with CLO. These findings are in keeping with a study by Parilla *et al.* [41], who also had age-matched controls. Not only could this group not show a difference in acid exposure between patients with severe oesophagitis and those with CLO, but similar results were found for basal sphincter pressure and oesophageal contractile amplitude for the two groups. Vaezi and Richter [42] also failed to find a statistically significant difference between all patients with oesophagitis and a group with uncomplicated CLO.

Singh *et al.* [43] found a correlation between the length of CLO and proximal oesophageal acid exposure.

There has been considerable interest in the possible role of duodenal contents in the pathogenesis of CLO and its complications. Conjugated bile acids in an acid environment, and unconjugated bile acids and trypsin in a neutral environment have been shown to be damaging to the oesophageal mucosa [44]. It is now possible to quantify duodenogastro-oesophageal reflux on a 24-hour ambulatory basis using a fibreoptic transnasal probe to detect bilirubin in refluxate (pp. 17–18). However, Vaezi and Richter [42] could not find greater duodenogastro-oesophageal reflux (DGOR) in patients with uncomplicated CLO than in those with oesophagitis without CLO. They also found that the DGOR paralleled acid reflux, and both decreased with omeprazole therapy [42,45]. They concluded that acid and duodenal contents could have a synergistic damaging role. Using the same technique, Caldwell *et al.* [46] found more DGOR in patients with CLO than in those with mild oesophagitis, but patients with severe oesophagitis were not evaluated.

Vaezi and Richter [47] also investigated patients with complicated CLO (stricture, ulcer and high-grade dysplasia) and found statistically sig-nificantly greater oesophageal acid exposure and DGOR compared with patients with CLO without complications. These findings are also compatible with a synergistic role for acid and duodenal contents in the pathogenesis of complications and with these being related to the amount of oesophageal exposure to refluxate.

Rarely, CLO may occur in an anacid environment years after a total gastrectomy [48], but simple oesophagitis is rare unless there is concomitant acid reflux (p. 20) [49].

In conclusion, it is not clear why some patients develop CLO. The pathophysiological changes in oesophageal motility, sphincter function, acid reflux and duodenogastro-oesophageal reflux in patients with uncomplicated CLO have not consistently been demonstrated to differ from those with severe erosive/ulcerative oesophagitis.

THE CANCER RISK

The evidence linking CLO to adenocarcinoma of the oesophagus and gastric cardia is overwhelming. Most cases of the former and many of the latter are associated with CLO [50–52]. Patients with CLO have about a 40-fold greater risk of adenocarcinoma than the general population [53]. Prospective studies of endoscopic surveillance have shown an incidence of about 1/100 patient years [53]. Squamous cell carcinoma of the oesophagus has also been linked to CLO. This is not a tumour of increasing incidence [52].

Adenocarcinoma of the oesophagus and cardia have an incidence increasing by 4–10% per year, which is a more rapid increase than that of any other malignancy in the Western world [54–58]. In line with these findings the incidence of CLO also appears to be rising: a fourfold increase between 1955 and 1973 and a 10-fold increase between 1963 and 1975 have been reported [59].

Despite the risk of adenocarcinoma, most patients with CLO die of other causes [60].

There have been reports of an increased risk of colon cancer in patients with CLO, but this has not been confirmed by others [26].

DYSPLASIA AND OTHER TUMOUR MARKERS

Dysplasia is defined as an unequivocal neoplastic transformation of the mucosa, which can give rise directly to an underlying invasive cancer and which is sometime the superficial part of a carcinoma [52]. It is classified as low-grade (LGD) or high-grade (HGD). Although invasive carcinoma can arise from either, it is much more likely to do so from HGD. LGD can be a reversible result of inflammation, e.g. oesophagitis [61].

There is considerable interobserver variation in the assessment of dysplasia, particularly for LGD, but less so for HGD. In one series there was nearly 90% agreement on HGD, but substantially less on LGD, despite slides being viewed by expert specialist histopathologists [62].

Most, if not all adenocarcinoma-associated CLO arises from HGD [52]. However, HGD may be patchy in distribution and therefore missed in surveillance biopsies [63]. If it is found on biopsy, at least one-third of patients will have an invasive carcinoma [64]. Most patients with HGD will progress to invasive carcinoma within 3 years [65]. Many authorities therefore recommend prophylactic oesophagectomy for HGD if the patient is otherwise fit.

Although HGD is undoubtedly the best marker of early or imminent invasive carcinoma other potential biochemical and molecular markers have been evaluated. By analogy with carcinoma of the stomach, greater sulphomucin expression (compared with sialomucin) in the CLO might be relevant to the development of malignancy, but its presence is so common in non-dysplastic CLO that it is probably not a useful marker for increased carcinoma risk [66]. However, it is conceivable that a reduction in sulphomucin expression resulting from treatment might indicate a reduced cancer risk [27].

Molecular markers of malignancy evaluated in CLO include EGF, c-erbB2, TGF-α and p53 [67]. Unfortunately most of these have proved insufficiently sensitive or specific for clinical use. p53 is perhaps the most promising. This is a tumour suppresser gene located on the short arm of chromosome 17. Mutation and deletion, which have been reported in a number of adenocarcinomas, result in accumulation of p53 protein, which is detectable by immunostaining of biopsy material. It is frequently found in CLO, HGD and adenocarcinoma, but has no advantage over assessing dysplasia.

Flow cytometry has been evaluated. This is a method of rapidly measuring the DNA content of cells. In a prospective study Reid *et al.* [68] followed 62 patients with CLO for a mean of 34 months. Nine of 13 with abnormal flow cytometry (aneuploidy or G2/tetraploidy) developed HGD, four of these also developing carcinoma, whereas none of 39 without abnormalities developed HGD or carcinoma. Menke-Pluymers *et al.* [69], however, could not relate ploidy to dysplasia, but G2/tetroploidy was found to be a risk factor independent of HGD for the development of carcinoma in patients under the age of 65 years. Fennerty *et al.* [70] also failed to show concordance between aneuploidy and dysplasia. Thus more data is required before flow cytometry can be recommended for routine assessment of biopsies from patients with CLO.

SURVEILLANCE FOR HGD AND CARCINOMA

A 50-year-old patient diagnosed as having CLO but with an otherwise normal life expectancy of 75 years has a one in four chance of developing adenocarcinoma. It may therefore seem logical to survey endoscopically patients with CLO regularly in the hope that early surgically curable carcinoma can be detected. There is no doubt that CLO-related carcinoma detected by surveillance has a much better prognosis than if it presents symptomaticaly – 85% compared with 20% respectively surviving up to 5 years of follow up in one series [71]. However, oesophagectomy is a major undertaking and clearly only patients who are acceptable surgical risks should be entered into surveillance programmes. The cost of surveillance must also be considered. The most recent UK study estimates this to be approximately £15 000 for male patients and £42 000 for females for every carcinoma detected (figures based on annual endoscopy with multiple biopsies) [72]. An estimate from the USA was $62 000 in 1988 [73].

Results of surveillance

Of three large prospective studies comprising 327 patients followed for a mean of four years, 15 developed carcinoma of whom 12 underwent surgical resection [23,72,74]. In one study [72] the results of surgery are not recorded, but of six patients in the other two series two died as a result of the operation and four appear to have been cured. One patient in one of the series [23] was not operated on because of coexisting carcinoma of the prostate from which he died 6 years later!

Thus there seems no doubt that endoscopic surveillance may detect asymptomatic cancer from which surgical cure can be expected, but the relatively long-term survivor who did not undergo oesophageal resection raises the question of the natural history and prognosis of surveillance-detected carcinoma.

The finding of HGD involves perhaps one of the most difficult decisions to face the clinician. It may be impossible to exclude a well differentiated invasive carcinoma in endoscopic biopsies as these do not usually contain adequate submucosal tissue. Although many favour prophylactic oesophagectomy, some patients may undoubtedly survive for several years without surgery [65].

Recommendations for surveillance

There is little conclusive data on which to base firm recommendations. The following is based on a working party report from the 1990 World Congress of Gastroenterology [26] and a study by Levine *et al.* [65].

If patients are physically fit enough to be potential candidates for oesophagectomy they should enter a regular endoscopic surveillance programme. At each endoscopy four quadrant biopsies, preferably with large forceps, should be taken every 2 cm from immediately below to immediately above the CLO and should be assessed by a histopathologist with particular expertise in this area. If there is no dysplasia biennial follow-up endoscopy is appropriate. If there is low-grade dysplasia a proton-pump inhibitor should be given for at least 3 months and the endoscopy should be repeated. If the dysplasia has resolved the patient should then undergo biennial endoscopy, but if it persists endoscopy should be repeated 6-monthly. If high-grade dysplasia is found surgery should be considered, or endoscopy with multiple biopsies should be repeated 6-monthly. If there is doubt about the changes of dysplasia from any endoscopy it should be repeated forthwith.

TREATMENT OF COLUMNAR-LINED OESOPHAGUS

As already pointed out, CLO *per se* does not cause symptoms. The usual goal of treatment of CLO is to induce a regression or ablation of the metaplastic columnar epithelium in the hope that this will reduce the chances of malignant transformation, but this remains unproven.

Drug therapy

H_2-receptor antagonists have been unsuccessful [75]. More recently the more powerful PPIs have been evaluated although none of those currently available have a product licence for this indication. A 30% regression in the linear extent of the CLO has been reported after 2 years

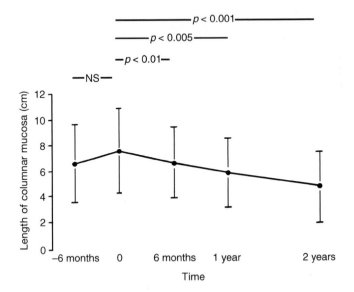

Figure 6.2 Linear regression of columnar-lined oesophagus with 2 years of treatment with omeprazole 40 mg daily. (Source: redrawn from reference 27, with permission of the publisher.)

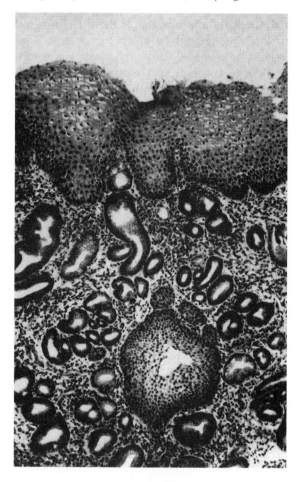

Figure 6.3 Macroscopic squamous island in columnar-lined oesophagus, showing squamous epithelialization of oesophageal gland duct following omeprazole therapy. (Source: from reference 27, with permission of the publisher.)

of continuous omeprazole 40 mg daily (Figure 6.2) [27], but continuing treatment up to 5 years did not produce further linear change [76]. Other evidence for regression included emergence of macroscopic and microscopic squamous islands within the CLO (each of which further increased from years 2 to 5), macroscopic squamous encroachment of the CLO at the squamocolumnar junction, and squamous metaplasia of the duct and gland tissue (Figure 6.3). In one of 16 patients the CLO appeared to regress completely both macroscopically and microscopically, while in another patient low-grade dysplasia, demonstrated in biopsies consistently up to year 3, was not found in any biopsy at years 4 and 5 [76].

It is now apparent that 40 mg of omeprazole daily may be insufficient to control acid reflux even if symptoms have resolved [77]. A recent study using 60 mg daily showed more than 50% reduction in the length of CLO after just 1 year of treatment [78]. Thus further studies using sufficient omeprazole to ensure complete control of acid reflux, based on pH monitoring, are needed.

The emergence and enlargement of squamous islands, but no linear regression, have been reported using omeprazole 20 mg daily and lansoprazole 60 mg daily [79,80].

Clearly, proton-pump inhibitors, at least in conventional doses, do not usually induce complete regression of CLO. Whether or not the partial control achieved will reduce the subsequent risk of malignancy has yet to be determined.

CLO ablation combined with acid suppression

Several endoscopic methods of CLO ablation have now been explored. These have all been used in conjunction with omeprazole. A report by Sampliner *et al.* [81] of the use of multipolar electrocoagulation achieved regression in 10 of 11 patients with regrowth of squamous epithelium over the treated area. Thermal laser ablation has given inconsistent results [82,83]. Berenson *et al.* [84] used an argon laser with substantial regression. These techniques need treatment to be repeated on several occasions to achieve full apparent regression. Biopsies have often shown the persistence of intestinal metaplasia beneath the new squamous epithelial skin. Whether or not the remaining abnormal tissue, no longer exposed to the presumed noxious refluxate, remains at risk of malignant transformation is unknown.

An alternative endoscopic method to thermal ablation is photodynamic therapy (PDT), again used in conjunction with omeprazole. The principle of PDT is that an administered photosensitizer selectively accumulates in neoplastic tissue. Application of light of an appropriate wavelength will activate the chemical and produce tissue necrosis. The technique is being used to treat a variety of tumours. Laukka and Wang [85] have treated mainly non-dysplastic CLO using haemoprotoporphyrin-derivative as a sensitizer. Substantial, but not complete regression was reported. Overholt and Panjehpour [86] used sodium porphimer as the photosensitizer in 36 patients with dysplasia (grade unspecified), 14 also having superficial carcinoma. Dysplasia was eliminated in 29 and malignancy in all. Complete regression of CLO was achieved in only 10. Strictures occurred in 21 patients, but were treated successfully by dilatation. Barr *et al.* [87] successfully used endogenously generated protoporphyrin IX as the photosensitizer to eradicate high-grade dysplasia in five patients. In each of these series columnar epithelium was found to persist beneath the new squamous skin.

Anti-reflux surgery

The results of anti-reflux surgery on CLO are inconsistent. Most carefully evaluated series have shown only minimal benefit [88]. A more recent study from Sagar *et al.* [89] reported regression in 24 of 56 patients, but progression in nine. Although the data are not given, the overall effect is not likely to have been statistically significant and the authors point out the difficulty in accurately assessing the length of CLO after surgery. However, the oesophageal pH recordings were more often normalized in the patients with regression, suggesting that the beneficial effect was real and dependent on the efficacy of the procedure in controlling reflux. Of interest was that regression was more likely in patients who had also undergone vagotomy. All of these series are uncontrolled and probably retrospectively analysed. The place of surgery will remain uncertain until a prospective randomized controlled trial is carried out.

Carcinoma can undoubtedly occur after successful anti-reflux surgery. In a recent series three of 112 patients developed adenocarcinoma during a median follow-up of 6.5 years [90].

POTENTIAL IMPACT OF NEW TECHNOLOGY

A number of recent developments could enhance the value of endoscopic surveillance and treatment of HGD/mucosal carcinoma. The techniques of magnification endoscopy combined with indigocarmine staining, and laser-induced fluorescent spectrometry could both improve the endoscopist's ability to locate areas of dysplasia for targeting biopsies (p. 62). In fact, biopsy might not even be necessary with the latter technique. If the early results of photodynamic therapy for treating high-grade dysplasia and mucosal carcinoma are confirmed these could transform management and would substantially 'move the goalposts' of who should enter surveillance programmes, as otherwise unfit patients could easily survive this form of treatment.

REFERENCES

1. Barrett NR. Chronic peptic ulcer of the oesophagus and 'oesophagitis'. *Br J Surg* 1950; **38**: 175–182.
2. Tileston W. Peptic ulcer of the esophagus. *Am J Med Sci* 1906; **132**: 240–265.
3. Allison PR, Johnstone AS. The oesophagus lined with gastric mucus membrane. *Thorax* 1953; **8**: 87–101.

4. Barrett NR. The lower esophagus lined by columnar epithelium. *Surgery* 1957; **41**: 881–894.
5. Moersch RN, Ellis FH, McDonald JR. Pathologic changes occurring in severe reflux esophagitis. *Surg Gynecol Obstet* 1959; **108**: 476–484.
6. Haywood J. The lower end of the oesophagus. *Thorax* 1961; **16**: 36–41.
7. Paull A, Trier JS, Dalton MD *et al*. The histologic spectrum of Barrett's esophagus. *N Engl J Med* 1976; **295**: 476–480.
8. Weinstein WM, Ippoliti AF. The diagnosis of Barrett's esophagus: goblets, goblets, goblets. *Gastrointest Endosc* 1996; **44**: 91–95.
9. Reid BJ, Weinstein WM. Barrett's esophagus and adenocarcinoma. *Annu Rev Med* 1987; **38**: 477–492.
10. Spechler SJ, Goyal RK. The columnar-lined esophagus, intestinal metaplasia, and Norman Barrett. *Gastroenterology* 1996; **110**: 614–621.
11. Hamilton SR, Smith RRL, Cameron JL. Prevalence and characteristics of Barrett's esophagus in patients with adenocarcinoma of the esophagus or esophagogastric junction. *Hum Pathol* 1998; **19**: 942–948.
12. Schnell TG, Sontag SJ, Chejfec G. Adenocarcinoma arising in tongues or short segments of Barrett's esophagus. *Dig Dis Sci* 1992; **37**: 137–143.
13. Spechler SJ, Zeroogian JM, Antonioli DA *et al*. Prevalence of metaplasia at the gastro-oesophageal junction. *Lancet* 1994; **344**: 1533–1536.
14. Johnston MH, Hammond AS, Laskin W, Jones DM. The prevalence and clinical characteristics of short segments of specialized intestinal metaplasia in the distal esophagus on routine endoscopy. *Am J Gastroenterol* 1996; **91**: 1507–1511.
15. Weston AP, Krmpotich P, Makdisi WF *et al*. Short segment Barrett's esophagus: clinical and histological features, associated endoscopic findings, and association with gastric intestinal metaplasia. *Am J Gastroenterol* 1996; **91**: 981–986.
16. Nandurkar S, Talley NJ, Martin CJ *et al*. Short segment Barrett's oesophagus: prevalence , diagnosis and associations. *Gut* 1997; **40**: 710–715.
17. Chalasani N, Wo JM, Hunter JG, Waring JP. Significance of intestinal metaplasia in different areas of the esophagus including esophagogastric junction. *Dig Dis Sci* 1997; **42**: 603–607.
18. Trudgill N J, Suvarna SK, Kapur KC, Riley SA. Intestinal metaplasia at the squamocolumnar junction in patients attending for diagnostic gastroscopy. *Gut* 1997; **41**: 585–589.
19. Cameron AJ. Epidemiology of columnar-lined esophagus and adenocarcinoma. *Gastroenterol Clin North Am* 1997; **26**: 487–494.
20. Cameron AJ, Lomboy CT. Barrett's esophagus: age, prevalence, and

extent of columnar epithelium. *Gastroenterology* 1992; **103**: 1241–1245.

21. Jochem VJ, Fuerst PA, Fromkes JJ. Familial Barrett's esophagus associated with adenocarcinoma. *Gastroenterology* 1992; **102**: 1400–1402.

22. Lomboy C, Cameron A, Carpenter H. Development of Barrett's esophagus: how long does it take? *Am J Gastroenterol* 1991; **86**: 1298.

23. Iftikhar SY, Janes PD, Steele RJC *et al.* Length of Barrett's oesophagus: an important factor in the development of dysplasia and adenocarcinoma. *Gut* 1992; **33**: 1155–1158.

24. Cooper BT, Barbezat GO. Barrett's oesophagus: a clinical study of 52 patients. *Q J Med* 1987; **62**: 97–108.

25. Johnson DA, Winters C, Spurling TJ *et al.* Esophageal acid sensitivity in Barrett's esophagus. *J Clin Gastroenterol* 1987; **9**: 23–27.

26. Dent J, Bremner CG, Collen MJ *et al.* Barrett's oesophagus. *J Gastroenterol Hepatol* 1991; **6**: 1–22.

27. Gore S, Healey CJ, Sutton R *et al.* Regression of columnar-lined (Barrett's) oesophagus with continuous omeprazole therapy. *Aliment Pharmacol Ther* 1993; **7**: 623–628.

28. Skinner D, Walther BC, Riddell RH *et al.* Barrett's esophagus: comparison of benign and malignant cases. *Ann Surg* 1983; **198**: 554–566.

29. Kim SL, Waring JP, Spechler *et al.* Diagnostic inconsistencies in Barrett's esophagus. *Gastroenterology* 1994; **107**: 945–949.

30. Woolf GM, Riddell RH, Irvine EJ, Hunt RH. A study to examine agreement between endoscopy and histology for the diagnosis of columnar-lined (Barrett's) esophagus. *Gastrointest Endosc* 1989; **35**: 541–544.

31. Canto MIF, Setrakian MHSS, Petras RE *et al.* Methylene blue selectively stains intestinal metaplasia in Barrett's esophagus. *Gastrointest Endosc* 1996; **44**: 1–7.

32. Stevens PD, Lightdale CJ, Green PHR *et al.* Combined magnification endoscopy with chromoendoscopy for the evaluation of Barrett's esophagus. *Gastrointest Endosc* 1994; **40**: 747–749.

33. Panjehpour M, Overholt BF, Vo-Dinh T *et al.* Endoscopic fluorescence detection of high-grade dysplasia in Barrett's esophagus. *Gastroenterology* 1996; **111**: 93–101.

34. Robey SS, Hamilton SR, Gupta PK, Erozan YS. Diagnostic value of cytopathology in Barrett's esophagus and associated carcinoma. *Am J Clin Pathol* 1988; **89**: 493–498.

35. Waxman I. Endosonography in columnar-lined esophagus. *Gastroenterol Clin North Am* 1997; **26**: 607–612.

36. Jankowski J. Gene expression in Barrett's mucosa: acute and chronic adaptive responses in the oesophagus. *Gut* 1993; **34**: 1649–1650.

37. Iascone C, DeMeester TR, Little AG *et al.* Barrett's esophagus: functional assessment, proposed pathogenesis and surgical therapy. *Arch Surg* 1983; **118**: 543–549.

38. Zaninotto G, DeMeester TR, Bremner CG *et al.* Esophageal function in patients with reflux-induced strictures and its relevance to surgical treatment. *Ann Thorac Surg* 1989; **47**: 362–370.

39. Gillen P, Keeling P, Byrne PJ *et al.* Barrett's oesophagus: pH profile. *Br J Surg* 1987; **74**: 774–776.

40. Neumann CS, Cooper PT. 24 hour ambulatory oesophageal pH monitoring in uncomplicated Barrett's oesophagus. *Gut* 1994; **35**: 1352–1355.

41. Parrilla P, Ortiz A, Martinez de Haro LF, Aguayojl Ramirez P. Evaluation of the magnitude of gastro-oesophageal reflux in Barrett's oesophagus. *Gut* 1990; **31**: 964–967.

42. Vaezi MF, Richter JE. Role of acid and duodenogastroesophageal reflux in gastroesophageal reflux disease. *Gastroenterology* 1996; **111**: 1192–1199.

43. Singh P, Taylor RH, Colin-Jones DG. Esophageal motor dysfunction and acid exposure in reflux esophagitis are more severe if Barrett's metaplasia is present. *Am J Gastroenterol* 1994; **89**: 349–356.

44. Kivilaakso E, Fromm D, Silen W. Effect of bile salts and related compounds on isolated esophageal mucosa. *Surgery* 1980; **87**: 280–285.

45. Champion G, Richter JE, Vaezi MF *et al.* Duodenogastroesophageal reflux: relationship to pH and importance in Barrett's esophagus. *Gastroenterology* 1994; **107**: 747–754.

46. Caldwell MTP, Lawlor P, Byrne PJ *et al.* Ambulatory oesophageal bile reflux monitoring in Barrett's oesophagus. *Br J Surg* 1995; **82**: 657–660.

47. Vaezi MF, Richter JE. Synergism of acid and duodenogastro-esophageal reflux in complicated Barrett's esophagus. *Surgery* 1995; **117**: 699–704.

48. Nishimaki T, Watanabe K, Suzuki T *et al.* Early esophageal adenocarcinoma arising in a short segment of Barrett's mucosa after total gastrectomy. *Am J Gastroenterol* 1996; **91**: 1856–1857.

49. Sears RJ, Champion G, Richter JE. Characteristics of partial gastrectomy patients with esophageal symptoms and duodenogastric reflux. *Am J Gastroenterol* 1995; **90**: 211–215.

50. Cameron AJ, Lomboy CT, Pera M, Carpenter HA. Adenocarcinoma of the esophagogastric junction and Barrett's esophagus. *Gastroenterology* 1995; **109**: 1541–1546.

51. Ireland AP, Clark GWB, DeMeester TR. Carcinoma of the cardia: role of short-segment Barrett's esophagus and columnar metaplasia. *Dis Esoph* 1996; **9**: 159–164.

52. Riddell RH. Early detection of neoplasia of the esophagus and gastroesophageal junction. *Am J Gastroenterol* 1996; **91**: 853–863.
53. Hudson N, Heading RC. Barrett's oesophagus: the role of surveillance and surgery. In: Farthing MJG, ed. *Clinical Challenges in Gastroenterology*. London: Dunitz, 1996: pp 29–41.
54. Blot WJ, Devesa SS, Kneller RW, Fraumeni JF. Rising incidence of adenocarcinoma of the esophagus and gastric cardia. *JAMA* 1991; **265**: 1287–1289.
55. Blot WJ, Devesa SS, Fraumeni JF. Continuing climb in rates of esophageal adenocarcinoma: an update. *JAMA* 1993; **270**: 1320.
56. Hesketh PJ, Clapp RW, Doos WG, Spechler SJ. The increasing frequency of adenocarcinoma of the esophagus. *Cancer* 1989; **64**: 526–530.
57. Powell J, McConkey CC. Increasing incidence of adenocarcinoma of the gastric cardia and adjacent sites. *Br J Cancer* 1990; **62**: 440–443.
58. Pera M, Cameron AJ, Trastek VF *et al.* Increasing incidence of adenocarcinoma of the esophagus and esophagogastric junction. *Gastroenterology* 1993; **104**: 510–513.
59. Wienbeck M, Barnert J. Epidemiology of reflux disease and reflux esophagitis. *Scand J Gastroenterol* 1989; **24**(Suppl 156); 7–13.
60. Van der Burg A, Dees J, Hop WCJ, van Blankenstein M. Oesophageal cancer is an uncommon cause of death in patients with Barrett's oesophagus. *Gut* 1996; **39**: 5–8.
61. Haggitt RC. Barrett's esophagus, dysplasia, and adenocarcinoma. *Hum Pathol* 1994; **25**: 982–993.
62. Reid BJ, Haggitt RC, Rubin CE *et al.* Observer variation in the diagnosis of dysplasia in Barrett's esophagus. *Hum Pathol* 1988; **19**: 166–178.
63. Cameron AJ, Carpenter HA. Barrett's esophagus, high-grade dysplasia, and early adenocarcinoma: a pathological study. *Am J Gastroenterol* 1997; **92**: 586–591.
64. Spechler SJ. Complications of gastroesophageal reflux disease. In: Castell DO, ed. *The Esophagus*. 2nd ed. Boston, MA: Little, Brown, 1995: pp 533–545.
65. Levine DS, Haggitt RC, Blount PL *et al.* An endoscopic biopsy protocol can differentiate high-grade dysplasia from early adenocarcinoma in Barrett's esophagus. *Gastroenterology* 1993; **105**: 40–50.
66. Jass JR. Mucin histochemistry of the columnar epithelium of the oesophagus: a retrospective study. *J Clin Pathol* 1981; **34**: 866–870.
67. Wright TA, Kingsnorth AN. Barrett's oesophagus and markers of malignant potential. *Eur J Gastroenterol Hepatol* 1994; **6**: 656–662.
68. Reid BJ, Blunt PL, Rubin CE *et al.* Flow-cytometric and histological progression to malignancy in Barrett's esophagus: prospective endoscopic surveillance of a cohort. *Gastroenterology* 1992; **102**: 1212–1219.

69. Menke-Pluymers MBE, Mulder AH, Hop WCJ *et al.* Dysplasia and aneuploidy as markers of malignant degeneration in Barrett's oesophagus. *Gut* 1994; **35**: 1348–1351.

70. Fennerty MB, Sampliner RE, Way D *et al.* Discordance between flow-cytometric abnormalities and dysplasia in Barrett's esophagus. *Gastroenterology* 1989; **97**: 815–820.

71. Peters JH, Clark GWB, Ireland AP *et al.* Outcome of adenocarcinoma arising in Barrett's oesophagus in endoscopically surveyed and non-surveyed patients. *J Thorac Cardiovasc Surg* 1994; **108**: 813–822.

72. Wright TA, Gray MR, Morris AI *et al.* Cost effectiveness of detecting Barrett's cancer. *Gut* 1996; **39**: 574–579.

73. Achkar E, Carey W. The cost of surveillance for adenocarcinoma complicating Barrett's esophagus. *Am J Gastroenterol* 1998; **83**: 291–294.

74. Hameeteman W, Tytgat GNJ, Houthoff HJ, van den Tweel JG. Barrett's esophagus: development of dysplasia and adenocarcinoma. *Gastroenterology* 1989; **96**: 1249–1256.

75. Sampliner RE, Garewal HS, Fennerty M, Aickin M. Lack of impact of therapy on extent of Barrett's esophagus in 67 patients. *Dig Dis Sci* 1990; **35**: 93–96.

76. Wilkinson SP. Biddlestone L, Gore S *et al.* Regression of columnar-lined (Barrett's) oesophagus with omeprazole: results of five years of continuous therapy. Submitted for publication, 1998.

77. Katzka DA, Castell DO. Successful elimination of reflux symptoms does not insure adequate control of acid reflux in patients with Barrett's esophagus. *Am J Gastroenterol* 1994; **89**: 989–991.

78. Malesci A, Savarino V, Zentilin P *et al.* Partial regression of Barrett's esophagus by long-term therapy with high-dose omeprazole. *Gastrointest Endosc* 1996; **44**: 700–705.

79. Neumann CS, Iqbal TH, Cooper BT. Long-term continuous omeprazole treatment of patients with Barrett's oesophagus. *Aliment Pharmacol Ther* 1995; **9**: 451–454.

80. Sampliner RE. Effective up to three years of high-dose lansoprazole on Barrett's esophagus. *Am J Gastroenterol* 1994; **89**: 1844–1848.

81. Sampliner RE, Fennerty B, Garewal HS. Reversal of Barrett's esophagus with acid suppression and multipolar electrocoagulation: preliminary results. *Gastrointest Endosc* 1996; **44**: 523–525.

82. Sampliner RE, Hixson LJ, Fennerty MB, Garewal HS. Regression of Barrett's esophagus by laser ablation in an anacid environment. *Dig Dis Sci* 1993; **38**: 365–368.

83. Luman W, Lessels AM, Palmer KR. Failure of Nd-YAG photocoagulation therapy as treatment for Barrett's oesophagus, a pilot study. *Eur J Gastroenterol Hepatol* 1996; **8**: 627–630.

84. Berenson MM, Johnson TD, Markowitz NR *et al.* Restoration of

squamous mucosa after ablation of Barrett's esophageal epithelium. *Gastroenterology* 1993; **104**: 1686–1691.

85. Laukka MA, Wang KK. Initial results using low-dose photodynamic therapy in the treatment of Barrett's esophagus. *Gastrointest Endosc* 1995; **42**: 59–63.

86. Overholt BF, Panjehpour M. Photodynamic therapy for Barrett's esophagus: clinical update. *Am J Gastroenterol* 1996; **91**: 1719–1723.

87. Barr H, Shepherd NA, Dix A *et al*. Eradication of high-grade dysplasia in columnar-lined (Barrett's) oesophagus by photodynamic therapy with endogenously generated protoporphyrin IX. *Lancet* 1996; **348**: 584–585.

88. Williamson WA, Ellis FH, Gibbs SP *et al*. Effect of anti-reflux operation on Barrett's mucosa. *Ann Thorac Surg* 1990; **49**: 537–541.

89. Sagar PM, Ackroyd R, Hosie KB *et al*. Regression and progression of Barrett's oesophagus after anti-reflux surgery. *Br J Surg* 1995; **82**: 806–810.

90. McDonald ML, Trastek VF, Allan MS *et al*. Barrett's esophagus: does an anti-reflux procedure reduce the need for endoscopic surveillance? *J Thorac Cardiovasc Surg* 1996; **111**: 1135–1140.

7

Gastro-oesophageal reflux – respiratory complications

The association between gastro-oesophageal reflux and respiratory disorders was firmly established in the 1960s [1,2]. In one study no less than 61% of 636 patients referred for anti-reflux surgery had respiratory symptoms [2]. The most common were cough and bronchitis. Many subsequent studies have confirmed these observations, with a prevalence of gastro-oesophageal reflux ranging from 33–90% in adults with a variety of respiratory disorders and 47–64% in children [3].

The spectrum of respiratory disorders associated with gastro-oesophageal reflux includes apnoea, sudden infant death syndrome, laryngitis, hoarseness, cough, nocturnal choking, pneumonia, bronchiectasis, fibrosis and asthma. It can be envisaged that each of these might be a direct mechanical/chemical effect of the refluxate on the particular tissue of the respiratory tract. That this can occur has been most convincingly shown by combined intratracheal and intra-oesophageal pH monitoring [4]. A vagal reflex bronchoconstriction initiated by acid in the distal oesophagus has also been proposed [5].

ASTHMA

Asthma is undoubtedly the most common potentially serious respiratory disorder associated with gastro-oesophageal reflux. Most research interest has therefore been focused on this association which has been evaluated from several different approaches. At least two-thirds of asthmatics have been reported to have reflux symptoms [6,7], abnormal acid reflux on the basis of pH monitoring has been found in up to 82% [8], while in a single study 39% had endoscopic oesophagitis with or without Barrett's metaplasia [9].

There are four possible ways in which asthma and gastro-oesophageal reflux might be associated.

- Gastro-oesophageal reflux might be secondary to drugs prescribed for treatment of the asthma.
- Gastro-oesophageal reflux might cause or exacerbate asthma.
- Asthma might cause or exacerbate gastro-oesophageal reflux.
- The two conditions might not be directly related to one another but share a common pathogenic mechanism.

Role of asthma medication

Theophyllines and β_2 agonists may impair gastro-oesophageal sphincter function [10,11], but these do not usually appear to have any significant effect in clinical usage [8,12,13].

Gastro-oesophageal reflux may cause/exacerbate asthma

The most obvious explanation for the association between reflux and asthma is that refluxed acid may trigger asthma, either by microaspiration or via vagal reflexes. However, the association between the two conditions does not necessarily indicate that one is consequent on the other. Indeed Ekström and Tibbling. [14,15], although recognizing the association, could not confirm daytime or nocturnal asthma to be preceded by gastro-oesophageal reflux.

If reflux does precipitate asthma the latter should be improved by effective anti-reflux therapy, either medical or surgical. Three double-blind placebo-controlled crossover trials of H_2-receptor antagonists have not shown anything other than a minimal benefit in respiratory measurements [16–18].

Two double-blind placebo-controlled crossover trials of omeprazole have now been conducted in patients with reflux and asthma. In the study of Ford *et al.* [19] omeprazole 20 mg daily was given for 4 weeks to 11 patients with reflux and asthma. Its use was not associated with improvement in asthma symptoms during the day or at night, respiratory function tests or bronchodilator usage. Meier *et al.* [20] used 40 mg of omeprazole daily for 6 weeks in an otherwise similar study. Of 15 patients they identified four in whom respiratory function tests improved by more than 20% with omeprazole treatment.

In an open study by Harding *et al.* [21] the dose of omeprazole was titrated against the results of oesophageal pH monitoring to ensure adequate acid suppression. Of the 30 patients enrolled, eight required more than 20 mg daily. Treatment was given for three months and 22 were reported to show an improvement in their asthma symptoms or peak expiratory flow rates (PEFRs). However, the PEFRs in these patients were not particularly reduced (379 l/m ± 30, compared with 262 l/m ± 86 in the study of Ford *et al.*). Furthermore the improvement in PEFR in the 'responders' was modest (to only 414 l/m ± 32), with many of this group showing only a minimal improvement. From their data it would appear the improvements in the responders may have been balanced by deteriorations in the non-responders with no overall statistically significant benefit, but this information was not provided. Of interest from their study was that when improvement did occur this showed a trend to be continuing at three months.

There are a number of uncontrolled surgical series reporting an impressive benefit of an anti-reflux procedure on asthma and other respiratory disorders [3], but objective data is often lacking. A study by Ruth *et al.* [22] could find objective evidence for improvement in respiratory function tests in only two of 13 asthmatics one year after successful fundoplication. A controlled trial by Larrain *et al.* [23] reported a better symptom score in patients treated surgically than in those treated by cimetidine or placebo. However, objective measurements of respiratory function were not given and the apparent improvement in the cimetidine group at 6 months was much higher than in other reported series. A preliminary report of another randomized trial of 73 patients showed that anti-reflux surgery substantially improved asthma, both symptomatically and objectively, compared with ranitidine or placebo [24].

What can be concluded from these studies? Despite several decades and numerous reports of the effects of acid suppression or surgery there is still no consistent convincing evidence to implicate gastro-oesophageal reflux as a major pathogenic factor in asthma, at least for the majority of patients. More prolonged randomized controlled trials of effective acid suppression and anti-reflux surgery with detailed objective assessments of respiratory function are needed. The presently available limited data does not exclude a contributory role in some patients.

Asthma may cause/exacerbate gastro-oesophageal reflux

This possible mechanism has rarely been considered. In one series the duration of asthma symptoms was longer than that of the symptoms of reflux [19]. Asthma will be characterized by markedly negative intra-thoracic pressures during inspiration. It is easy to envisage these changes provoking acid reflux, particularly as asthmatics often have a reduced lower oesophageal sphincter pressure [8].

It is possible that a vicious cycle might develop between gastro-oesophageal reflux and asthma, with one exacerbating the other.

Gastro-oesophageal reflux and asthma share a common pathogenic mechanism

There is evidence that both gastro-oesophageal reflux [25] and asthma [26] may be associated with a vagal nerve dysfunction, which could account for the more than chance association of both conditions.

COUGH, LARYNGITIS, HOARSENESS AND GLOBUS

Gastro-oesophageal reflux has been reported in 10–20% of patients with otherwise unexplained cough [27,28] and in many patients a bout of coughing can be shown to be preceded by an episode of reflux [29]. Treatment of the reflux may cure the cough [27,30,31]. However, cough can also precipitate reflux. In one study cough was twice as likely to precede reflux as vice versa [32].

A variety of other 'laryngeal symptoms', including hoarseness, globus and throat-clearing, have also been linked to gastro-oesophageal reflux. The subject has recently been extensively reviewed by Fraser [33]. Some 55–79% of patients with hoarseness and 10–65% with globus presenting to ENT departments have been reported to show abnormal gastro-oesophageal reflux on oesophageal pH monitoring. In one study 30 of 97 patients with hoarseness, a burning sensation in the pharynx or globus had abnormal acid reflux [34].

Patients with these associations often have 'posterior laryngitis', which is characterized by erythema, nodularity, plaques and contact ulcers [33], but these findings are not specific for reflux-associated laryngeal disorders [34].

The possible mechanism to explain the link between reflux and laryngeal problems, as with asthma, includes both the direct effects of refluxed material and reflex mechanisms. Some support is given to the reflux component by Jacob *et al.* [35]. They investigated 40 patients with proven reflux who had a variety of laryngeal symptoms including hoarseness, cough, globus, frequent throat-clearing or sore throat. They found a greater prevalence of acid reflux in the proximal oesophagus than in controls. More recently, Shaker *et al.* [36], using three-site ambulatory pharyngeal/oesophageal pH monitoring, confirmed a link between pharyngeal acid reflux and posterior laryngitis.

It is of interest that in many of these series with reflux and respiratory symptoms the patients have often not experienced the usual symptoms of reflux, i.e. heartburn and/or regurgitation.

REFERENCES

1. Kennedy JH. 'Silent' gastroesophageal reflux: an important but little known cause of pulmonary complications. *Dis Chest* 1962; **42**: 42–45.

2. Urschel HC, Paulson DL. Gastroesophageal reflux and hiatal hernia: complications and therapy. *J Thorac Cardiovasc Surg* 1967; **53**: 21–32.
3. Sontag SJ. Pulmonary complications of gastroesophageal reflux. In: Castell DO, ed. *The Esophagus*. 2nd ed. Boston, MA: Little, Brown, 1995: pp 555–570.
4. Jack CIA, Calverley PMA, Donnelly RJ *et al*. Simultaneous tracheal and oesophageal pH measurements in asthmatic patients with gastro-oesophageal reflux. *Thorax* 1995; **50**: 201–204.
5. Mansfield LE, Stein MR. Gastroesophageal reflux and asthma, a possible reflex mechanism. *Ann Allergy* 1978; **41**: 224–226.
6. O'Connell S, Sontag SJ, Miller T *et al*. Asthmatics have a high prevalence of reflux symptoms regardless of the use of broncho-dilators. *Gastroenterology* 1990; **98**: A97.
7. Field SK, Underwood M, Brant R, Cowie RL. Prevalence of gastroesophageal reflux symptoms in asthma. *Chest* 1996; **109**: 316–322.
8. Sontag S, O'Connell S, Khandelwal S *et al*. Most asthmatics have gastroesophageal reflux with or without broncho-dilator therapy. *Gastroenterology* 1990; **99**: 613–620.
9. Sontag SJ, Schnell TG, Miller TQ *et al*. Prevalence of oesophagitis in asthmatics. *Gut* 1992; **33**: 872–876.
10. Berquist WE, Rachelefsky GS, Kadden M *et al*. Effect of theophylline on gastroesophageal reflux in normal adults. *J Allergy Clin Immunol* 1981; **67**: 407–411.
11. DiMarino AJ, Cohen S. Effect of an oral β_2-adrenergic agonist on lower esophageal sphincter pressure in normals and in patients with achalasia. *Dig Dis Sci* 1982; **27**: 1063–1066.
12. Hubert D, Gaudric M, Guerre J *et al*. Effect of theophylline on gastroesophageal reflux in patients with asthma. *J Allergy Clin Immunol* 1988; **81**: 1168–1175.
13. Sontag S, O'Connell S, Khandelwal S *et al*. Effect of positions, eating and broncho-dilators on gastroesophageal reflux in asthmatics. *Dig Dis Sci* 1990; **35**: 849–856.
14. Ekström T, Tibbling L. Gastro-oesophageal reflux and triggering of bronchial asthma: a negative report. *Eur J Respir Dis* 1987; **71**: 177–180.
15. Ekström T, Tibbling L. Gastro-oesophageal reflux and nocturnal asthma. *Eur Respir J* 1988; **1**: 636–638.
16. Goodall RJR, Earis JE, Cooper DN *et al*. Relationship between asthma and gastro-oesophageal reflux. *Thorax* 1981; **36**: 116–121.
17. Ekström T, Lindgren BR, Tibbling L. Effects of ranitidine treatment on patients with asthma and a history of gastro-oesophageal reflux: a double blind cross-over study. *Thorax* 1981; **44**: 19–23.
18. Nagel RA, Brown P, Perks WH *et al*. Ambulatory pH monitoring of

gastro-oesophageal reflux in 'morning dipper' asthmatics. *Br Med J* 1988; **296**: 1371–1373.

19. Ford GA, Oliver PS, Prior JS *et al*. Omeprazole in the treatment of asthmatics with nocturnal symptoms of gastro-oesophageal reflux: a placebo-controlled cross-over study. *Postgrad Med J* 1994; **70**: 350–354.

20. Meier JH, McNally PR, Punja M *et al*. Does omeprazole improve respiratory function in asthmatics with gastroesophageal reflux? A double-blind, placebo-controlled cross-over study. *Dig Dis Sci* 1994; **39**: 2127–2133.

21. Harding SM, Richter JE, Guzzo MR *et al*. Asthma and gastroesophageal reflux: acid suppressive therapy improves asthma outcome. *Am J Med* 1996; **100**: 395–405.

22. Ruth M, Bake B, Sandberg N *et al*. Pulmonary function in gastroesophageal reflux disease – effect of reflux controlled by fundoplication. *Dis Esoph* 1994; **7**: 268–275.

23. Larrain A, Carrasco E, Galleguillos F *et al*. Medical and surgical treatment of nonallergic asthma associated with gastroesophageal reflux. *Chest* 1991; **99**: 1330–1335.

24. Sontag SJ, O'Connell S, Khandelwal S *et al*. Anti-reflux surgery in asthmatics with reflux improves pulmonary symptoms and function. *Gastroenterology* 1990; **98**: A128.

25. Ogilvie AL, James PD, Atkinson M. Impairment of vagal function in reflux oesophagitis. *Q J Med* 1985; **54**: 61–74.

26. Morrison JFJ, Pearson SB, Dean HG. Parasympathetic nervous system in nocturnal asthma. *Br Med J* 1988; **296**: 1427–1429.

27. Irwin RS, Curley FJ, French CL. Chronic cough. The spectrum and frequency of causes, key components and of the diagnostic evaluation, and outcome of specific therapy. *Am Rev Respir Dis* 1990; **141**: 640–647.

28. Pratter MR, Bartter T, Akers S, DuBois J. An algorithmic approach to chronic cough. *Ann Intern Med* 1993; **119**: 977–983.

29. Patterson WG, Murat BW. Combined ambulatory esophageal manometry and dual-probe pH-metry in evaluation of patients with chronic unexplained cough. *Dig Dis Sci* 1994; **39**: 1117–1125.

30. Waring JP, Lacayo L, Hunter J *et al*. Chronic cough and hoarseness in patients with severe gastroesophageal reflux disease. Diagnosis and response to therapy. *Dig Dis Sci* 1995; **40**: 1093–1097.

31. Johnston BT, Gideon RM, Castell DO. Excluding gastroesophageal reflux disease as a cause of chronic cough. *J Clin Gastroenterol* 1996; **22**: 168–169.

32. Laukka MA, Cameron AJ, Schei AJ. Gastroesophageal reflux and chronic cough: which comes first? *J Clin Gastroenterol* 1995; **19**: 100–104.

33. Fraser AG. Gastro-oesophageal reflux and laryngeal symptoms. *Aliment Pharmacol Ther* 1994; **8**: 265–272.
34. Wilson JA, White A, von Haacke M P *et al.* Gastroesophageal reflux and posterior laryngitis. *Ann Otol Rhinol Laryngol* 1989; **98**: 405–410.
35. Jacob P, Kahrilas PJ, Herzon G. Proximal esophageal pH-metry in patients with reflux laryngitis. *Gastroenterology* 1991; **100**: 305–310.
36. Shaker R, Milbrath M, Ren J *et al.* Esophagopharyngeal distribution of refluxed gastric acid in patients with reflux laryngitis. *Gastroenterology* 1995; **109**: 1575–1582.

8

Achalasia

Achalasia is a condition of the oesophagus characterized by failure of both peristalsis and lower oesophageal sphincter relaxation. It has a reported incidence of 0.5–1/100 000/year, affects males and females equally and usually presents between the ages of 30 and 60 years [1,2].

In most cases the cause is unknown, but a similar condition may occur secondary to malignancy, usually at the oesophagogastric junction ('pseudoachalasia').

Achalasia has a striking similarity to the oesophageal involvement in Chagas' disease, a condition prevalent in South America and caused by *Trypanosoma cruzi* but characterized by multiple visceral organ disease.

A rare condition presenting in childhood is associated with alacrima and adrenocortical insufficiency [3].

PATHOLOGY AND PATHOPHYSIOLOGY

Pathological changes in the lower oesophageal sphincter and oesophageal body of resected specimens consist of an intense chronic inflammatory infiltrate in the myenteric plexus together with loss of ganglion cells and focal replacement of neurones by collagen [4,5]. The inhibitory neurones of the sphincter are particularly affected. Their chief neurotransmitter substance is nitric oxide and nitric oxide synthetase has been found to be markedly reduced in the sphincter in achalasia [6].

Autoantibodies to the myenteric plexus have been described [7,8]. This finding, together with the chronic inflammatory infiltrate suggests at least a component of autoimmune damage, but the trigger factor is unknown. Previous reports of a possible association with measles or herpes infection [9,10] have not been confirmed using PCR techniques [11,12].

Apparently typical achalasia has been described following long-standing gastro-oesophageal reflux, a condition with an almost diametrically opposite pathophysiology [13]. The authors have drawn attention to the fact that vagal dysfunction has been described in both achalasia [14] and reflux [15] and that they might therefore be linked in some way. However, reflux affects perhaps 10% of the population. A chance association is therefore also possible. Of additional interest is a group of patients recently described in a retrospective analysis who had preceding symptoms of heartburn that ceased, as might be anticipated, by the development of dysphagia due to achalasia [16].

The neuromuscular abnormalities of achalasia may extend to the upper oesophageal sphincter [17,18], stomach [19] and gallbladder [20]. The possible overlap with spastic motility disorders of the oesophagus is discussed in Chapter 9.

CLINICAL FEATURES AND COMPLICATIONS

Dysphagia is by far the most common symptom. However, regurgitation, weight loss, chest pain, heartburn and cough are all common (Table 8.1) [21,22].

Dysphagia is painless and for both liquids as well as solids. The degree of weight loss will depend on the duration of the disease and the severity of the dysphagia. The regurgitated food may be noticed to be totally undigested and/or acidic-tasting, the latter being due to fermentation. Dysphagia occurs particularly while recumbent and may result in cough and other pulmonary complications. Chest pain is of a variable nature, but may be severe and mimic ischaemic heart pain (Chapter 10).

Heartburn is a particularly important symptom that may lead to an incorrect and delayed diagnosis and even to inappropriate anti-reflux surgery [23]. Occasionally it may be due to gastro-oesophageal reflux and, as already pointed out, this may precede achalasia. However, other more likely explanations for heartburn include stagnation with fermentation of ingested food [24], oesophageal retention of ingested acidic drinks, and

Table 8.1   Symptoms in achalasia (data from reference 21, based on nearly 2000 patients in 14 published studies, with permission of the publisher)

Symptoms	Mean % of patients with symptoms
Dysphagia	97
Regurgitation	75
Weight loss	58
Chest pain	43
Heartburn	36
Cough	30

the fact that both oesophageal distension and spasm may be interpreted as 'heartburn' (Chapter 10).

Other rarer complications of achalasia include bezoar of the oesophagus, oesophagobronchial and oesophagopericardial fistulae and perforation [22]. Involvement of the upper oesophageal sphincter with failure of relaxation may result in an impaired belch reflex with gross air trapping in the oesophagus, which has resulted in acute respiratory obstruction [25,26] and may be corrected by cricopharyngeal myotomy [27].

Squamous cell carcinoma is well recognized in achalasia. Its reported prevalence and incidence range widely, many of the studies being retrospective. In a prospective study of 195 patients undergoing surveillance endoscopy and followed for at least 10 years an incidence of 3.4/1000/year was found [28]. Columnar-lined (Barrett's) oesophagus, a well-known precursor of adenocarcinoma, may result from reflux consequent to therapeutic sphincter rupture [29].

DIAGNOSIS

Unfortunately, the diagnosis of achalasia is often made only many years after the initial symptoms manifest themselves [21,22]. Specific investigations include radiology, manometry and scintigraphy.

Radiology

In advanced achalasia a plain chest X-ray may reveal a widened mediastinum with a fluid level, while an upright straight abdominal X-ray may lack the normal gastric air bubble. A barium swallow will show the oesophagus to be widely dilated with a 'bird beak' distal tapering (Figure 8.1). Fluoroscopy will demonstrate absent peristalsis. However, in early disease there may be no dilatation and tertiary contractions may be noted. Prospective studies of the value of contrast radiology have reported a correct diagnosis in 22 of 33 [2] and 15 of 37 patients [30], with a variety of misdiagnoses in the others.

Manometry

Manometry is the gold standard for diagnosis. The important abnormalities to swallowing are complete or partial failure of lower oesophageal sphincter relaxation and aperistalsis of the smooth muscle segment of the oesophageal body. The resting intra-oesophageal pressure is characteristically higher than the intragastric pressure (a reversal of the norm) and basal sphincter pressure is often elevated. Of these four changes Castell considers only the absence of peristalsis to be essential for

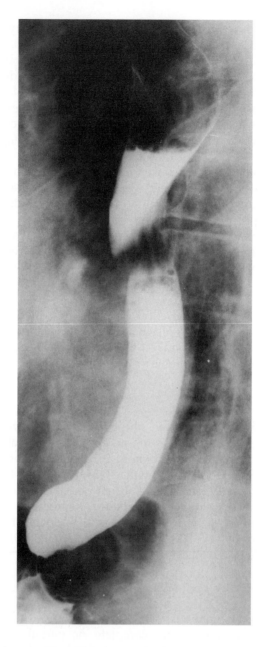

Figure 8.1   Barium swallow of patient with advanced achalasia showing widely dilated oesophagus and tightly closed oesophogastric sphincter.

diagnosis [31]. Although the body of the oesophagus may be atonic a variety of types of pressure wave may be seen, including simultaneous contractions that are of low amplitude and long duration in the dilated oesophagus. If these are repetitive and of high amplitude (> 60 mmHg) the condition is referred to as 'vigorous achalasia' [31]. Propagated pressure waves may occasionally be seen after successful balloon dilatation of the sphincter [32].

It must be added that a recent 24-hour ambulatory manometric study showed that patients with achalasia may have propagated peristalsis, though less commonly than in healthy controls, the individual contraction waves being of lower amplitude and longer duration [33].

Despite the well-defined criteria the manometric diagnosis is **not** always straightforward. Technical problems relating to accurate sphincter measurements are discussed elsewhere (Chapter 19) and it may be particularly difficult to pass the recording catheter through the sphincter in achalasia. Up to 30% of patients may show complete sphincter relaxation although the episodes are of short duration [34]. Propagated peristalsis in the upper, striated muscle part of the oesophagus may lead to confusion. Aperistalsis of the distal oesophagus may be confused with scleroderma. Vigorous achalasia may be confused with diffuse oesophageal spasm.

Scintigraphy

Radionuclide transit scintigraphy, particularly using solid meals in the upright posture, may show delayed distal oesophageal emptying [35], but failed to diagnose achalasia in 12 out of 37 patients in one recent study [30]. It should be regarded as complementary to manometry for assistance in the diagnosis of difficult cases rather than as an alternative.

PSEUDOACHALASIA

Tumour infiltration of the lower oesophageal sphincter, particularly by adenocarcinoma, may cause an achalasia-like clinical presentation with similar oesophageal manometric changes. Other tumours, including some remote from the sphincter, may also cause pseudoachalasia [21]. It is therefore imperative that any patient with suspected achalasia undergoes endoscopy for careful inspection and biopsy of the sphincter region to try to eliminate a malignant cause. Endoscopic ultrasound might also prove to be particularly useful in excluding tumour.

TREATMENT

Smooth muscle relaxants are of only very limited value [21]. Bougie dilatation is of only transient benefit. More definitive and usually very effective are mechanical methods of disrupting the sphincter, by either balloon inflation or surgical myotomy. Recently botulinum toxin has been used to paralyse the sphincter, with encouraging preliminary results.

Balloon rupture

Some 80–90% of patients respond favourably to balloon rupture [21,22]. The technique is straightforward. Under benzodiazepine sedation a guidewire is positioned endoscopically in the stomach. The endoscope is removed, and the balloon is passed over the guidewire and inflated, usually under fluoroscopic control. Because of retained food debris in the oesophagus the patient may need to have been kept on fluids only for a few days. In the most severe cases oesophageal lavage with a wide-bore tube is necessary. For the latter group it may be preferable to carry out the procedure under general anaesthetic so the airway can be adequately protected during lavage.

There has been little comparative scientific evaluation of protocols for balloon dilatation, particularly with regard to the size of balloon, inflation pressure and duration of inflation. Most of the following is therefore based on uncontrolled studies, hearsay, experience and a little common sense. The now most commonly used balloons are the fixed-size polytuff devices (Rigiflex), which are available in 30, 35 and 40 mm diameters. Balloon diameter is probably more important than inflation pressure. Most endoscopists use pressures of 2–20 psi (100–1000 mmHg) for 30–60 seconds [22]. There is less likelihood of perforation or subsequent gastro-oesophageal reflux with smaller balloons. It is therefore preferable to start with the smallest balloon and repeat the procedure a few weeks later with a larger balloon if necessary. On average patients require 1.4 dilatations before satisfaction is achieved [21].

The chief risk of balloon dilatation is perforation, with a reported prevalence of 0–15% [22]. There is no agreed protocol for routine checking immediately after the procedure. Some recommend a meticulous endoscopy followed by a contrast swallow. Others would merely advise careful observation for chest pain, other distress and fever. Certainly it is prudent to admit the patient overnight. If perforation does occur it can usually be managed conservatively, but surgery should not be delayed if indicated (p. 54).

Surgical myotomy

The short-term results of open surgical myotomy are similar to those reported for balloon rupture [22]. The procedure can be carried out through the abdomen or the chest. More recently, laparoscopic [36], thorascopic [37] and endoscopic [38] approaches have been described.

Assessment of efficacy of balloon rupture or surgical myotomy

There is no agreed protocol for assessing the results of sphincter disruption, but techniques include clinical evaluation, measuring the diameter of the cardia on contrast swallow, manometry and radionuclide scintigraphy [39,40]. In the setting of clinical trials objective assessments are clearly necessary, but in routine practice a clinical assessment is probably adequate. However, if there is recurrence of dysphagia a full re-evaluation is necessary as this does not necessarily indicate a recurrence of achalasia and may be due to a peptic stricture, or even carcinoma, secondary to treatment-induced reflux (see below).

Gastro-oesophageal reflux following balloon rupture or surgical myotomy

Disruption of the sphincter inevitably exposes the patient to gastro-oesophageal reflux. The risk is often said to be greatest following surgical myotomy [22], but this is not borne out by a large meta-analysis [41]. In one series abnormal reflux could be demonstrated in nearly 40% of patients after 1 year, whether they had been treated by balloon dilatation or by surgical myotomy, but not all were symptomatic [42]. In another series of 176 patients mostly treated by balloon dilatation and followed for up to 27 years, there were 47 (27%) cases of reflux [43]. To avoid reflux some surgeons routinely carry out a fundoplication at the time of myotomy, but with the advent of proton-pump inhibitors this may no longer be necessary. The additional anti-reflux procedure may itself result in dysphagia [44].

A benign stricture may complicate treatment-induced reflux. Of 66 cases treated by balloon dilatation and followed for at least 10 years this occurred in eight of 18 who developed reflux [45].

As stated above, columnar-lined oesophagus may complicate sphincter disruption. This was found in four of 46 patients followed for a mean period of 13 years [29].

Long-term results of balloon rupture or surgical myotomy

There are few long-term analyses of results with either treatment. The limited data available indicate that with either balloon rupture or open myotomy about one-third of the patients show a clinically relevant deterioration at 10 years, which rises to two-thirds by 20 years [45,46]. Before further surgical treatment is contemplated a detailed re-evaluation is necessary to ascertain the cause of failure so that appropriate procedures can be offered to the patient, some even requiring oesophagectomy [46].

Botulinum toxin

Botulinum toxin inhibits acetylcholine release from nerve terminals. Its successful use in achalasia by injection into the lower oesophageal sphincter was first described by Pasricha *et al.* [47] with improvement usually apparent within a few days. A subsequent randomized controlled trial by the same group showed a 90% response and two-thirds of the patients remained in remission at 1 year [48]. Another randomized controlled trial confirmed the efficacy of botulinum toxin, but seven out of eight patients required a second injection to sustain remission [49]. In the latter study patients initially receiving placebo saline injection showed no improvement in symptom score, reduction in lower oesophageal sphincter pressure or oesophageal retention as measured by scintigraphy. They were subjected to balloon dilatation, the results of which were almost identical at 1 month to the group who had received botulinum toxin.

A subsequent study by Pasricha *et al.* [50] followed 31 patients for a mean of $2\frac{1}{2}$ years; 28 improved immediately with a mean duration of clinical response of 1.3 years. A better response was found in patients over the age of 50.

In most of the above studies a total dose of 100 u of toxin as Botox was injected. However, different preparations are available. It is essential to check dose equivalence before use.

Which treatment?

Until some 3 years ago the usually recommended first-line treatment would have been balloon rupture, with one or two further attempts if necessary. In the minority of patients in whom this was unsuccessful referral for an open surgical myotomy would then have been appropriate. It would not have been unreasonable to have chosen surgical myotomy as the first line of treatment for younger patients, as they do less well with balloon rupture [51,52]. Failures of surgical myotomy could be offered balloon rupture as a second line of treatment. In expert hands the two techniques appear to be of comparable efficacy, with a similar complication rate, but myotomy, with the more prolonged hospital stay, is more expensive. One randomized controlled trial of balloon dilatation versus surgical myotomy suggested the superiority of the latter, but balloon dilatation was only applied for 20 seconds or less, with a very low success rate of only approximately 60% [53].

The use of botulinum toxin and laparoscopic/thorascopic myotomy may change the future. The risk of perforation from balloon rupture is not present with botulinum injection. Some of the arguments against open myotomy, such as length of hospital stay, may be nullified by the newer techniques. Only large prospective randomized controlled trials will provide the necessary answers. However, for the elderly frail patient or the patient in whom there is doubt about the diagnosis of achalasia, botulinum toxin would appear to be the treatment of choice.

REFERENCES

1. Mayberry JF, Atkinson M. Studies of the incidence and prevalence of achalasia in the Nottingham area. *Q J Med* 1985; **56**: 451–456.
2. Howard PJ, Maher L, Pryde A *et al*. Five year prospective study of the incidence, clinical features, and diagnosis of achalasia in Edinburgh. *Gut* 1992; **33**: 1011–1015.
3. Allgrove J, Clayden GS, Grant DB, Macauley JC. Familial glucocorticoid deficiency with achalasia of the cardia and deficient tear production. *Lancet* 1978; **i**: 1284–1286.
4. Goldblum JR, Whyte RI, Orringer MB, Appelman HD. Achalasia. A morphologic study of 42 resected specimens. *Am J Surg Pathol* 1994; **18**: 327–337.
5. Goldblum JR, Rice TW, Richter JE. Histopathologic features of esophagomyotomy specimens from patients with achalasia. *Gastroenterology* 1996; **111**: 648–654.
6. Mearin F, Mourelle M, Guarner F *et al*. Patients with achalasia lack nitric oxide synthase in the gastro-oesophageal junction. *Eur J Clin Invest* 1993; **23**: 724–728.
7. Singaram C, Sweet MA, Belcaster GM *et al*. A novel autoantibody exists in patients with esophageal achalasia. *Gastroenterology* 1994; **106**: A566.
8. Verne GN, Sallustio JE, Eaker EY. Anti-myenteric neuronal antibodies in patients with achalasia. A prospective study. *Dig Dis Sci* 1997; **42**: 307–313.
9. Jones DB, Mayberry JF, Rhodes J, Munro J. Preliminary report of an association between measles virus and achalasia. *J Clin Pathol* 1983; **36**: 655–657.
10. Robertson CS, Martin BA, Atkinson M. Varicella-zoster virus DNA in the oesophageal myenteric plexus in achalasia. *Gut* 1993; **34**: 299–302.
11. Niwamoto H, Okamoto E, Fujimoto J *et al*. Are human herpes viruses or measles virus associated with esophageal achalasia? *Dig Dis Sci* 1995; **40**: 859–864.
12. Birgisson S, Galinski MS, Goldblum JR *et al*. Achalasia is not associated with measles or known herpes and human papilloma viruses. *Dig Dis Sci* 1997; **42**: 300–306.
13. Smart HL, Mayberry JF, Atkinson M. Achalasia following gastro-oesophageal reflux. *J R Soc Med* 1986; **79**: 71–73.

14. Woolam GL, Mayer FT, Ellis FH. Vagal nerve function in achalasia of the esophagus. *Surg Forum* 1967; **18**: 362–365.
15. Ogilvie AL, James PD, Atkinson M. Impairment of vagal function in reflux oesophagitis. *Q J Med* 1985; **54**: 61–74.
16. Spechler SJ, Souza RF, Rosenberg SJ *et al*. Heartburn in patients with achalasia. *Gut* 1995; **37**: 305–308.
17. Jones B, Donner MW, Rubesin SE *et al*. Pharyngeal findings in 21 patients with achalasia of the esophagus. *Dysphagia* 1987; **2**: 87–92.
18. Becker DJ, Castell DO. Acute airway obstruction in achalasia. *Gastroenterology* 1989; **97**: 1323–1326.
19. Eckart VF, Krause J, Bolle D. Gastrointestinal transit and gastric acid secretion in patients with achalasia. *Dig Dis Sci* 1989; **34**: 665–671.
20. Annese V, Caruso N, Accadia L *et al*. Gallbladder function and gastric liquid emptying in achalasia. *Dig Dis Sci* 1991; **36**: 1116–1120.
21. Birgisson S, Richter JE. Achalasia: what's new in diagnosis and treatment? *Dig Dis* 1997; **15**(Suppl 1): 1–27.
22. Wong RKH, Maydonovitch CL. Achalasia. In: Castell DO, ed. *The Esophagus*. 2nd ed. Boston, MA: Little, Brown, 1995: pp 219–245.
23. Ellis FH, Crozier FE, Gibb SP. Reoperative achalasia surgery. *J Thorac Cardiovasc Surg* 1986; **92**: 859–865.
24. Smart HL, Foster PN, Evans DF *et al*. 24 hour oesophageal acidity in achalasia before and after pneumatic dilatation. *Gut* 1987; **28**: 883–887.
25. Massey BT, Hogan WJ, Dodds WJ, Dantas RO. Alteration of the upper esophageal sphincter belch reflex in patients with achalasia. *Gastroenterology* 1992; **103**: 1574–1579.
26. Dunlop SP, Travis SPL. Achalasia presenting as acute stridor. *Eur J Gastroenterol Hepatol* 1997; **9**: 1125–1128
27. Campbell KL, Logi JRC, Munro A. Cricopharyngeus myotomy for upper airway obstruction in achalasia. *Br J Surg* 1995; **82**: 1668–1669.
28. Meijssen MAC, Tilanus HW, van Blankenstein M *et al*. Achalasia complicated by oesophageal squamous cell carcinoma: a prospective study in 195 patients. *Gut* 1992; **33**: 155–158.
29. Jaakkola A, Reinikainen P, Ovaska J, Isolauri J. Barrett's esophagus after cardiomyotomy for esophageal achalasia. *Am J Gastroenterol* 1994; **89**: 165–169.
30. Stacher G, Schima W, Bergmann H *et al*. Sensitivity of radionuclide bolus transport and videofluoroscopic studies compared with manometry in the detection of achalasia. *Am J Gastroenterol* 1994; **89**: 1484–1488.
31. Troshinsky MB, Castell DO. Achalasia. In: Castell DO, Castell JA, eds. *Esophageal Motility Testing*. 2nd ed. Norwalk, CT: Appleton & Lange, 1994: pp 109–121.
32. Vantrappen G, Agg HO, Janssens J *et al*. Achalasia, diffuse esophageal

spasm, and related motility disorders. *Gastroenterology* 1979; **76**: 450–457.

33. Di Martino N, Bortolotti M, Izzo G *et al*. 24-hour esophageal ambulatory manometry in patients with achalasia of the esophagus. *Dig Dis Sci* 1997; **10**: 121–127.

34. Katz PO, Richter JE, Cowan R, Castell DO. Apparent complete lower esophageal sphincter relaxation in achalasia. *Gastroenterology* 1986; **90**: 978–983.

35. Holloway RH, Krosin G, Lange RC *et al*. Radionuclide esophageal emptying of a solid meal to quantitate results of therapy in achalasia. *Gastroenterology* 1983; **84**: 771–776.

36. Shimi S, Nathanson LK, Cushieri A. Laparoscopic cardiomyotomy in achalasia. *J R Coll Surg Edin* 1991; **36**: 152–154.

37. Pellegrini CA, Leichter R, Patti M *et al*. Thorascopic esophageal myotomy in the treatment of achalasia. *Ann Thorac Surg* 1993; **56**: 680–682.

38. Ortega JA, Madureri V, Perez L. Endoscopic myotomy in the treatment of achalasia. *Gastrointest Endosc* 1980; **26**: 8–10.

39. Robertson CS, Hardy JG, Atkinson M. Quantitative assessment of the response to therapy in achalasia of the cardia. *Gut* 1989; **30**: 768–773.

40. Parker DR, Swift GL, Adams H *et al*. Radionuclide esophageal transit studies in achalasia before and after balloon dilatation. *Dis Esoph* 1996; **9**: 42–44.

41. Ferguson MK. Achalasia – current evaluation and therapy. *Ann Thorac Surg* 1991; **52**: 336–342.

42. Shoenut JP, Duerksen D, Yaffe CS. A prospective assessment of gastroesophageal reflux before and after treatment of achalasia patients: pneumatic dilatation versus transthoracic limited myotomy. *Am J Gastroenterol* 1997; **92**: 1109–1112.

43. Dakkak M, Cox JGC, Bennett JR. Gastroesophageal reflux as a complication of achalasia therapy. *Gastroenterology* 1997; **112**: A96.

44. Ellis RH. Oesophagomyotomy for achalasia: a 22-year experience. *Br J Surg* 1993; **80**: 882–885.

45. Dakkak M, Bennett JR. 10-Year follow-up after forceful balloon dilatation of achalasia. *Gastroenterology* 1997; **112**: A97.

46. Malthaner RA, Todd TR, Miller L, Pearson FG. Long-term results in surgically managed esophageal achalasia. *Ann Thorac Surg* 1994; **58**: 1343–1347.

47. Pasricha PJ, Ravich WJ, Hendrix TR *et al*. Treatment of achalasia with intrasphincteric injection of botulinum toxin. A pilot trial. *Ann Intern Med* 1994; **121**: 590–591.

48. Pasricha PJ, Ravich WJ, Hendrix TR *et al*. Botulinum toxin for the treatment of achalasia. *N Engl J Med* 1995; **322**: 774–778.

49. Annese V, Basciani M, Perri F *et al*. Controlled trial of botulinum toxin

injection versus placebo and pneumatic dilatation in achalasia. *Gastroenterology* 1996; **111**: 1418–1424.

50. Pasricha PJ, Rai R, Ravich WJ *et al.* Botulinum toxin for achalasia: long-term outcome and predictors of response. *Gastroenterology* 1996; **110**: 1410–1415.

51. Robertson CS, Fellowes IW, Mayberry JF *et al.* Choice of therapy for achalasia in relation to age. *Digestion* 1998; **40**: 244–250.

52. Eckardt VF, Aignherr C, Bernhard G. Predictors of outcome in patients with achalasia treated by pneumatic dilatation. *Gastroenterology* 1992; **103**: 1732–1736.

53. Csendes A, Braghetto I, Burdiles P, Csendes P. Comparison of forceful dilatation and esophagomyotomy in patients with achalasia of the esophagus. *Hepatogastroenterology* 1991; **38**: 502–505.

9

Other oesophageal motility disorders

DIFFUSE OESOPHAGEAL SPASM, NUTCRACKER OESOPHAGUS, HYPERTENSIVE LOWER OESOPHAGEAL SPHINCTER, NON-SPECIFIC OESOPHAGEAL MOTILITY DISORDER

The terms diffuse oesophageal spasm (DOS), nutcracker oesophagus (NO), hypertensive lower oesophageal sphincter (HLOS), and non-specific oesophageal motility disorder (NSOMD) refer to manometric changes and should not necessarily be regarded as definitive clinical entities. They are sometimes referred to collectively as spastic oesophageal motility disorders. They characteristically affect the smooth muscle part of the oesophagus, i.e. the mid and lower thirds. They have been found particularly in patients presenting with chest pain and/or dysphagia. The detailed manometric findings are discussed below but, in brief, in response to wet swallows, DOS is characterized by simultaneous contractions of the entire oesophagus interspersed with normally propagated peristalsis, NO by abnormally high amplitude, but normally propagated contractions, and HLOS by an abnormally high basal sphincter pressure. NSOMD is characterized by abnormalities that are insufficient for one of these 'diagnoses'.

There is considerable overlap between each of these and one may evolve into another. Some 50% of patients with HLOS may also have NO [1], while the initial manometric diagnosis of DOS changed in no fewer than 50% of patients followed for a mean of $3\frac{1}{2}$ years in one series [2]. The changing pattern of abnormalities has also been shown by 24-hour ambulatory motility recording, the diagnosis with the latter completely agreeing with the findings of stationary manometry in only 51% of 108 patients [3]. Thus the findings on stationary manometry of DOS, NO, HLOS or NSOMD should perhaps be regarded as manifestations of wider oesophageal muscle dysfunction that may lead to the symptoms of dysphagia and/or chest pain. A specific clinical diagnosis should be reserved for those patients in whom symptoms have unequivocally been linked to manometric findings on ambulatory testing [3–6].

Achalasia is sometimes included with the above abnormalities within the same spectrum of motility disorders. Cases of DOS and NO have been described as evolving into vigorous achalasia or achalasia [7–10], but this is unusual [2]. The histological and ultrastructural changes to nerve fibres described in achalasia have not been found in diffuse oesophageal spasm [11].

The spastic oesophageal motility disorders can present at any age, but particularly in middle life. Dysphagia is characteristically to both liquids and solids. Chest pain is often swallow-induced, but can mimic ischaemic heart pain (Chapter 10). A number of patients have underlying gastro-oesophageal reflux [12]. Others have psychiatric disorders (especially depression, anxiety and somatization) – 84% in one series compared with 31% and 33% for two control groups [13]. Not surprisingly, therefore, symptoms are often worse at times of stress.

Manometric and radiological changes [14,15]

Diffuse oesophageal spasm
This is the least common of the group. Essential for the diagnosis is that at least 10% of 5 ml wet swallows are followed by simultaneous oesophageal contractions, with intermittent normal peristalsis. Other non-diagnostic findings include repetitive contractions, sometimes with three or more peaks, high-amplitude contractions (> 180 mmHg), prolonged contractions (> 6 s) and incomplete relaxation of, or hypertensive, lower oesophageal sphincter.

Radiologically the findings are of segmental spasm, or a rosary bead or corkscrew appearance.

Nutcracker oesophagus
The average distal peristaltic amplitude of 10 wet swallows must exceed 180 mmHg, but can be as high as 400 mmHg. Peristalsis is normally conducted.

Hypertensive lower oesophageal sphincter
The basal pressure of the sphincter exceeds 45 mmHg, relaxes to swallowing, but the latter may be incomplete.

Non-specific oesophageal motility disorders
A variety of changes may occur including non-propagated contractions, triple peaks, retrograde contractions, low-amplitude contractions

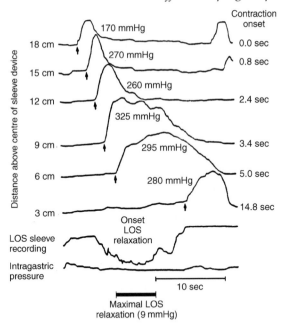

Figure 9.1 This patient with manometric criteria of nutcracker oesophagus and hypertensive lower oesophageal sphincter (pressure > 60 mmHg) complained of dysphagia that was relieved by anti-reflux therapy. (Source: redrawn from reference 12, with permission of the publisher.)

(< 30 mmHg), prolonged peristaltic waves (> 6 s) and isolated incomplete sphincter relaxation. A high percentage of these patients have abnormal gastro-oesophageal reflux, particularly in the supine posture [16].

Treatment

Numerous smooth muscle relaxants have been used for the treatment of both the dysphagia and pain of spastic oesophageal motility disorders, including nitrates and calcium-channel blockers. Very few randomized controlled trials have been carried out [13]. Treatment is therefore largely by trial and error, but the results are usually at best mediocre. Treatment of associated gastro-oesophageal reflux, if present, can be dramatically beneficial (Figure 9.1) [12,17]. These patients often do not give a classical history of reflux, the dysphagia and/or chest pain being the only symptoms [16–18]. Nitrates and calcium-channel blockers may, of course, exacerbate reflux.

Psychotropic drugs and behaviour therapy are often useful when there is a coexisting psychiatric diagnosis [13].

Pneumatic dilatation and surgical myotomy have been described, but before they are undertaken it is essential to exclude gastro-oesophageal reflux. Balloon dilatation of the oesophageal body, avoiding the lower oesophageal sphincter, using the 30 mm or 35 mm Rigiflex polytuff balloon improved symptoms in about 50% of patients in one study [19]. In another, for patients who had both diffuse oesophageal spasm and sphincter dysfunction, balloon dilatation of the sphincter improved dysphagia in eight of nine patients [20]. A long surgical myotomy may also be effective [19]. This can be carried out thorascopically [21]. More recently, injection of botulinum toxin into the lower oesophageal sphincter for a variety of spastic oesophageal motility disorders has been reported to be beneficial [22].

FAILURE OF SECONDARY PERISTALSIS AND REDUCED OESOPHAGEAL TRACTION FORCES DURING PRIMARY PERISTALSIS

These two manometric disorders have recently been described in patients with otherwise unexplained dysphagia. Their clinical importance remains to be established.

Secondary peristalsis is the progressive propagated oesophageal contraction occurring in the absence of swallowing. It is usually triggered by oesophageal distension, either by a food bolus not cleared by primary peristalsis or by refluxate from the stomach. Secondary peristalsis may in fact be more important than primary peristalsis in clearing a swallowed food bolus [23]. Schoeman and Holloway [24] have shown that secondary peristalsis is best evaluated by rapidly injecting 10 ml of water or air into the mid-oesophagus. In an assessment of 30 patients with non-obstructive dysphagia six of nine with normal primary peristalsis had defective secondary peristalsis. In the other 21 patients defective peristalsis was found in nine of 11 with diffuse oesophageal spasm and eight of 10 with non-specific oesophageal motility disorders. Thus defective secondary peristalsis might be an important cause for dysphagia in non-obstructive patients with normal standard manometry and also contribute to dysphagia in those with other motility disorders.

Williams *et al.* [25] have devised an intra-oesophageal catheter for measurement of traction forces during primary peristalsis. Of 12 patients with dysphagia of otherwise unknown cause (all patients had a normal barium swallow, endoscopy and stationary manometry) six had reduced traction forces despite normal-amplitude peristalsis recorded manometrically.

CRICOPHARYNGEAL DYSPHAGIA

The cricopharyngeus muscle is the main component of the upper oesophageal sphincter and is functionally integrated with the inferior pharyngeal constrictor muscle above and the cervical oesophagus below. It is approximately 1 cm long. It contracts during inspiration to prevent air entering the oesophagus. Its tonicity is increased by stress and reduced by sleep [12].

Defective opening of the cricopharyngeus muscle is a relatively common cause of dysphagia, especially in the elderly and in association with a variety of neurological and muscular disorders, including stroke, parkinsonism, motor neuron disease, myasthenia gravis and muscular dystrophy [26]. For the latter groups the cricopharyngeal muscular dysfunction is part of a more widespread problem also affecting the tongue, mouth and remainder of the pharynx.

The abnormal cricopharyngeus may show evidence of a restrictive myopathy, with muscle fibre degeneration and fibrous replacement, which are likely to reduce compliance and opening [27]. The condition is sometimes, perhaps inappropriately, referred to as upper oesophageal sphincter achalasia. The underlying pathological mechanisms are quite different from those found in achalasia of the cardia. Failure of relaxation of the cricopharyngeus may also be the underlying mechanism for the development of a pharyngeal pouch, although the link is controversial [28]. Defective relaxation of the cricopharyngeus has also been described in association with gastro-oesophageal reflux, but again the significance is uncertain [28].

The presenting symptom is usually high dysphagia, choking and pulmonary aspiration, as well as those of any associated underlying neurological/muscular disease. Radiologically the condition is characterized by a posterior indentation ('bar') in the barium column. Standard manometry is not suitable for diagnosis, circumferentially sensing transducers being necessary [29].

Dysphagia can often be improved substantially be cervical myotomy if the abnormality is largely confined to the cricopharyngeus and not part of a more widespread neuropathy/myopathy [30]. The procedure may result in aspiration in patients with underlying gastro-oesophageal reflux [12], but this is probably unusual [30].

REFERENCES

1. Freidin N, Traube M, Mittal RK *et al*. The hypertensive lower esophageal sphincter. *Dig Dis Sci* 1989; **34**: 1066–1067.
2. Achem SR, Benjamin S. Esophageal dysmotility (spastic dysmotility).

In: Castell DO, ed. *The Esophagus*. 2nd ed. Boston, MA: Little, Brown, 1995: pp 247–268.

3. Stein HJ. Clinical use of ambulatory 24-hour esophageal motility monitoring in patients with primary esophageal motor disorders. *Dysphagia* 1993; **8**: 105–111.

4. Janssens J, Vantrappen G, Ghillebert G. 24-hour recording of esophageal pressure and pH in patients with non-cardiac chest pain. *Gastroenterology* 1986; **90**: 1978–1984.

5. Richter JE, Castell DO. 24 hour-ambulatory oesophageal motility monitoring: how should motility data be analysed? *Gut* 1989; **30**: 1040–1047.

6. Barham CP, Gotley DC, Fowler A *et al*. Diffuse esophageal spasm: diagnosis by ambulatory 24 hour manometry. *Gut* 1997; **41**: 151–155.

7. Kramer P, Harris LD, Donaldson RM. Transition from symptomatic diffuse spasm to cardiospasm. *Gut* 1967; **8**: 115–119.

8. Vantrappen G, Agg HO, Janssens J *et al*. Achalasia, diffuse esophageal spasm and related motility disorders. *Gastroenterology* 1979; **76**: 450–457.

9. Anggiansah A, Brigh NF, McCullagh M *et al*. Transition from nutcracker esophagus to achalasia. *Dig Dis Sci* 1990; **35**: 1162–1166.

10. Howard PJ, Maher L, Pryde A *et al*. Five year prospective study of the incidence, clinical features, and diagnosis of achalasia in Edinburgh. *Gut* 1992; **33**: 1011–1015.

11. Friesen DL, Henderson RD, Hanna W. Ultrastructure of the esophageal muscle in achalasia and diffuse esophageal spasm. *Am J Clin Pathol* 1983; **79**: 319–325.

12. Kahrilas PJ. Esophageal motility disorders: pathogenesis, diagnosis, treatment. In: Champion MC, Orr WC, eds. *Evolving Concepts in Gastrointestinal Motility*. Oxford: Blackwell, 1966: pp 15–45.

13. Richter JE, Bradley LC. Psychophysiological interactions in esophageal diseases. *Sem Gastrointest Dis* 1996; **7**: 169–184.

14. Richter JE. Diffuse esophageal spasm. In: Castell DO, Castell JA, eds. *Esophageal Motility Testing*. 2nd ed. Norwalk, CT: Appleton & Lange, 1994: pp 122–134.

15. Castell DO. The nutcracker esophagus, the hypertensive lower esophageal sphincter and non-specific esophageal motility disorders. In: Castell DO, Castell JA, eds. *Esophageal Motility Testing*. 2nd ed. Norwalk, CT: Appleton & Lange, 1994: pp 135–147.

16. Leite LP, Johnston BT, Barrett J *et al*. Ineffective esophageal motility (IEM). The primary finding in patients with nonspecific esophageal motility disorder. *Dig Dis Sci* 1997; **42**: 1859–1865.

17. Achem SR, Kolts BE, Wears R *et al*. Chest pain associated with nutcracker esophagus: a preliminary study of the role of gastroesophageal reflux. *Am J Gastroenterol* 1993; **88**: 187–192.

18. Bancewicz J, Osugi H, Marples M. Clinical implications of abnormal oesophageal motility. *Br J Surg* 1987; **74**: 416–419.
19. Irving JD, Owen WJ, Linsell J *et al*. Management of diffuse esophageal spasm with balloon dilatation. *Gastrointest Radiol* 1992; **17**: 189–192.
20. Ebert EC, Ouyang A, Wright SH *et al*. Pneumatic dilatation in patients with symptomatic diffuse esophageal spasm and lower esophageal sphincter dysfunction. *Dig Dis Sci* 1983; **28**: 481–485.
21. Shimi SM, Nathanson LK, Cushieri A. Thorascopic long oesophageal myotomy for a nutcracker oesophagus: initial experience of a new surgical approach. *Br J Surg* 1992; **79**: 533–536.
22. Miller LS, Parkman HP, Schiano TD *et al*. Treatment of symptomatic nonachalasia esophageal motor disorders with botulinum toxin injection at the lower esophageal sphincter. *Dig Dis Sci* 1996; **41**: 2025–2031.
23. Dent J, Holloway RH. Esophageal motility and reflux testing. State-of-the-art and clinical role in the twenty-first century. *Gastroenterol Clin North Am* 1996; **25**: 51–73.
24. Schoeman MN, Holloway RH. Secondary oesophageal peristalsis in patients with nonobstructive dysphagia. *Gut* 1994; **35**: 1523–1528.
25. Williams D, Thompson DG, Marples M *et al*. Diminished oesophageal traction forces with swallowing in gastro-oesophageal reflux disease and in functional dysphagia. *Gut* 1994; **35**: 165–171.
26. Ekberg O, Wahlgren L. Dysfunction of pharyngeal swallowing: a cineradiographic investigation of 854 dysphageal patients. *Acta Radiol Diagn* 1985; **26**: 389–395.
27. Cook IJ, Blumbergs P, Cash K *et al*. Structural abnormalities of the cricopharyngeus muscle in patients with pharyngeal (Zenker's) diverticulum. *J Gastroenterol Hepatol* 1992; **7**: 556–562.
28. Ekberg O. Cricopharyngeal disorders. In: Bouchier IAD, Allan RN, Hodgson HJF, Keighley MRB, eds. *Gastroenterology, Clinical Science and Practice*. 2nd ed. Philadelphia, PA: WB Saunders, 1993: pp 43–56.
29. Castell JA, Castell DO. Upper esophageal sphincter and pharyngeal function and oropharyngeal (transfer) dysphagia. *Gastroenterol Clin North Am* 1996; **25**: 35–50.
30. Lerut T, Coosemans W, Cuypers P *et al*. The pharyngoesophageal segment: cervical myotomy as therapeutic principle for pharyngoesophageal disorders. *Dis Esoph* 1996; **9**: 22–32.

10

Chest pain of uncertain cause

Chest pain in patients who are found to have normal coronary angiography is an enormous clinical problem in terms of the number of patients, an often poor understanding of the mechanisms involved, and limited effective treatments available. Although the prognosis in terms of life expectancy is excellent [1,2], many patients remain chronically incapacitated by their symptoms and often continue to believe they have serious cardiac disease years later even after normal coronary angiography [2,3] or a positive diagnosis of an oesophageal disorder [4]. They are frequently referred between several specialists and usually undergo extensive expensive investigations. The condition has been estimated to cost $750 000 000 annually in the USA [5].

There are many causes of chest pain. Pleural, pericardial, musculoskeletal and chest wall disorders are usually easily diagnosed clinically, but most patients referred for specialist consultations are initially suspected of having ischaemic heart disease. If coronary angiography is normal and the other causes listed above have been excluded the condition is sometimes referred to as non-cardiac chest pain. However, as there is sometimes evidence for a cardiac source of the pain this term may be inappropriate. In the present text the term chest pain of uncertain cause (CPUC) will be used. Oesophageal causes are also now well recognized, as is the role of psychological/psychiatric factors.

SYMPTOMS AND THEIR PERCEPTION BY PATIENT AND PHYSICIAN

A careful history will often help to distinguish between cardiac and oesophageal causes of anterior chest pain. A crushing/constricting retrosternal discomfort radiating into the neck or arms that is reproduced by exercise with rapid relief on resting is suggestive of ischaemic heart pain. Symptoms suggestive of an oesophageal cause include retrosternal burning, relief by antacids, relationship to meals, nocturnal pain, regurgitation, dysphagia and odynophagia. Unfortunately the symptom overlap may be considerable and patients who have both proven ischaemic heart disease and gastro-oesophageal reflux are often unable to identify correctly the cause of individual episodes of pain [6]. The situation is further complicated by the fact that exercise may induce gastro-oesophageal reflux [7], although this is probably an uncommon cause of exertional chest pain [8]. Cardiologists and gastroenterologists are similarly often unable to make an accurate clinical diagnosis [9]. The difficulty in differentiating the origin of pain is not surprising in view of the shared sensory neural pathways from the heart and oesophagus.

The cerebral 'processing' of information may be different in patients with CPUC. A group with angina-like chest pain and normal coronary angiography had abnormal cerebral evoked potentials to balloon distension of the oesophagus compared with control subjects. These were of lower amplitude, of lower quality score and had longer latencies [10].

HEART

There are several cardiac causes for chest pain in patients with angiographically normal coronary arteries. Coronary artery spasm in the absence of atheromatous disease may cause angina [11]. Other causes include 'syndrome X' and increased cardiac pain perception.

In the 1970s it became recognized that some patients with exercise-induced angina and typical ischaemic ECG changes have angiographically normal coronary arteries. Collectively these patients are often referred to as having 'syndrome X' [12], but this is undoubtedly a heterogeneous group of conditions [13]. A subgroup of probably fewer than 30% may indeed have myocardial ischaemia as a cause for their pain, as evidenced by increased cardiac lactate production and an abnormal thallium scan [14]. These patients can legitimately be referred to as having 'microvascular angina'.

The myocardial ischaemia associated with microvascular angina may be due to endothelial dysfunction in that acetylcholine-induced endothelial-dependent dilatation of the coronary arteries has been shown to be defective [15]. This abnormality is probably widespread in that endothelial dysfunction of the brachial artery has also been demonstrated [16].

As a group, patients with syndrome X are often post-menopausal women with demonstrable oestrogen deficiency. Their response to conventional anti-anginal therapy is often poor [13,14].

There have been several demonstrations of increased pain perception in patients with CPUC. Shapiro *et al.* [17] provoked the patient's pain simply by manipulation of the catheter in the atrium or by rapid intra-atrial injection of saline. Cannon *et al.* [18], investigating 36 patients with normal coronary arteries, could provoke the pain in 31 by pacing at only 5 beats/min higher than the pre-existing heart rate. In 20 of the patients it was provoked by infusion of contrast into the left coronary artery. These manoeuvres caused pain in only two out of 42 patients with proven coronary artery disease. Others have demonstrated provocation of the pain by intravenous injection of adenosine [19] or dipyridamole [20].

OESOPHAGUS

Oesophageal causes of chest pain include gastro-oesophageal reflux and motility disorders. It may be of relevance in the context of a possible generalized endothelial dysfunction present in patients with microvascular angina (see above) that the pain associated with oesophageal motility disorders might also have an ischaemic basis [21].

Some 40–60% of patients with chest pain in whom ischaemic heart disease has been excluded have an oesophageal abnormality that **could** explain the pain. Methods of investigation include provocation tests, stationary oesophageal manometry and ambulatory pH and/or manometry.

Provocation tests

The most commonly used tests to provoke the patient's pain have been the acid perfusion test (APT), edrophonium infusion and inflation of an intra-oesophageal balloon.

In the APT, 0.1 N hydrochloric acid is instilled into the mid-oesophagus to assess whether this provokes the patient's pain (Chapter 19). Similarly pain may be provoked by rapid intravenous infusion of edrophonium 80 μg/kg. Curiously a positive APT does not mean that the patient's pain is due to acid reflux while a positive edrophonium test, which causes enhanced oesophageal contraction, does not necessarily indicate that the pain is due to oesophageal spasm [5,22]. Despite the lack of precise specificity of these tests, they have good specificity for demonstrating an oesophageal source of the pain.

A meta-analysis [22] showed the APT to be positive in 31% of 805 patients with CPUC (12 studies). For the edrophonium test 25% of 792 patients were positive (13 studies). When both tests were used 40% of 662 were positive (11 studies).

Balloon distension has demonstrated increased oesophageal

sensitivity in patients with CPUC. A balloon is positioned 10 cm above the lower oesophageal sphincter and inflated by 1 ml increments to 10 ml. Of 351 patients reported in five studies [22] the patient's usual pain was provoked in 22%. Furthermore it occurred at a lower inflation volume than when pain was provoked in the relatively few control subjects. These results are analogous to findings in irritable bowel syndrome [23].

Stationary manometry

Oesophageal motility disorders have frequently been found during stationary manometry. In a meta-analysis of 1624 patients with CPUC 39% were found to have an abnormality, of which 42% were nutcracker oesophagus, 25% non-specific oesophageal motility disorder, 12% diffuse oesophageal spasm, 16% hypertonic lower oesophageal sphincter and 11% achalasia, with more than one disorder in some patients [5]. However, in most instances the patients did not experience pain during the investigation. It cannot therefore be concluded that these abnormalities are in any way related to the patient's pain.

Ambulatory pH and/or oesophageal manometry

The advent of 24-hour continuous ambulatory monitoring has permitted a much more accurate assessment of the significance of acid reflux and oesophageal motility disorders in the pathogenesis of CPUC. If the pain occurs immediately following an oesophageal event with a frequency more than would be expected by chance alone it is a reasonable assumption that the event may have caused the pain (Chapter 19). This is in contrast to the provocation tests, which merely identify the oesophagus as a probable source of the pain.

Such 24-hour pH recordings have shown acid reflux to be the commonest oesophageal cause for CPUC. From several studies the pain and acid reflux show concordance in approximately 50% of such patients [24–27]. As with gastro-oesophageal reflux with a classical presentation, at least one-half of these patients do not have endoscopic oesophagitis [9].

Combined pH/motility monitoring has again shown the importance of acid reflux. In a meta-analysis of eight studies comprising 321 patients with CPUC, reflux alone preceded the patient's usual pain in 18%, motility disorders were related in 11%, and both in 9% [22]. The motility disorders were usually of a non-specific nature, not as clearly defined as in the stationary motility studies. In this same meta-analysis 64% of 261 patients in seven of the studies were reported to have experienced their pain during the investigation. It must be added that only 45% of 629 pain episodes in seven of the studies were related to an abnormal oesophageal event.

PSYCHOLOGICAL/PSYCHIATRIC FACTORS AND HYPERVENTILATION

In an analysis of 365 patients in seven studies 65% had a specific psychological/psychiatric diagnosis as assessed by structured interviews [28]. The most common are panic disorder, anxiety, depression, somatization and high levels of neuroticism [28,29]. More than one diagnosis is often present. Associated symptoms include inappropriate respiratory symptoms, palpitations, nausea, abdominal distension, tingling, dizziness and lethargy [30]. It has been pointed out that with the possible exception of panic disorder the prevalence of these abnormalities is similar to those reported in non-ulcer dyspepsia, irritable bowel syndrome and chronic fatigue syndrome [28,31]. The prevalence of all of these abnormalities is consistently higher than in control subjects or those with proven ischaemic heart disease [28,29,31]. Reduced coping mechanisms and spouse reinforcement have also been described [32] and there is sometimes a history of physical or sexual abuse [33].

Hyperventilation has long been recognized as a cause for cardiac-type chest pain [34]. Bass and colleagues have shown that patients with CPUC and hyperventilation, the latter evidenced by failure of the end tidal P_{CO_2} to rise during or immediately after an exercise stress ECG, are those most likely to have a high score for panic, anxiety and depression [30,35]. They have suggested that routine measurement of end tidal P_{CO_2} during an exercise ECG might identify patients who are most likely to have a psychological/psychiatric diagnosis rather than a cardiac disorder. These patients often complain of inappropriate symptoms of breathlessness, e.g. at rest, during minimal exertion or emotion, air hunger and suffocation. Interestingly, the chest pain associated with hypocapnia and normal coronary angiograms was found more likely to be 'typical cardiac' than atypical [35].

SUMMARY OF PATHOPHYSIOLOGICAL STUDIES

A number of demonstrated abnormalities might account for chest pain experienced by patients with angiographically normal coronary arteries. These include microvascular angina, gastro-oesophageal reflux and oesophageal motility disorders. In addition, a high proportion of these patients have an underlying psychological/psychiatric diagnosis and enhanced thoracic visceral sensitivity to a variety of stimuli. When these apparently diverse abnormalities have all been sought in the same patients more than one has often been found [36].

APPROACH TO THE PATIENT WITH CPUC

Once ischaemic heart disease and obvious pleural, pericardial, musculo-skeletal and chest wall causes have been excluded, the management of a patient with chest pain is often difficult and unrewarding. It may be appropriate during the cardiac evaluation to measure end expiratory Pco_2 to identify patients with hyperventilation/hypocapnia who are more likely to have an underlying psychiatric diagnosis [30,35]. As gastro-oesophageal reflux is a common and potentially treatable cause appropriate investigations should be performed. Although oesophageal provocation tests are easily carried out they do not prove reflux to be the cause of the pain. This can best be achieved by 24-hour pH monitoring with evidence for a correlation between the patient's symptoms and episodes of acid reflux. Preliminary reports show that omeprazole is more effective than placebo if the pain has been shown to be associated with reflux [37], but there are no randomized controlled trials of patients with CPUC as a group. A daily dose of 40 mg should be given and it may be reasonable to give a therapeutic trial without prior pH monitoring. Endoscopy will only confirm a diagnosis of reflux in a minority of patients. If the patient's symptoms seem to be temporarily related to a demonstrated spastic oesophageal motility disorder, as shown by ambulatory motility testing, most clinicians try nitrates, hydralazine or calcium-channel blockers, but results from randomized controlled trials have been disappointing [31].

If acid reflux is not deemed to be the cause of the patient's pain a structured psychological/psychiatric assessment should be made, which might reveal unsuspected abnormalities that may respond to appropriate treatment, particularly for depression. The results of studies using cognitive treatment have been variable [37–40]. A randomized double-blind controlled trial of imipramine 50 mg at night resulted in a 50% reduction in episodes of chest pain but the benefit was independent of the patient's psychological/psychiatric profile, suggesting that the mechanism was through a visceral analgesic effect [36].

Not infrequently all of these measures fail and, as already pointed out, patients may remain chronically disabled. Continuing chest pain was still present in 74% of 46 patients after a mean follow-up of 11.4 years after negative coronary angiograms, particularly in those with an underlying specific psychological/psychiatric diagnosis [2].

REFERENCES

1. Kemp HG, Vokonas PS, Cohn PF, Gorlin R. The anginal syndrome associated with normal coronary arteriograms: report of a six year experience. *Am J Med* 1973; **54**: 735–742.

2. Potts SG, Bass CM. Psychosocial outcome and use of medical resources in patients with chest pain and normal or near-normal coronary arteries. A long-term follow-up study. *Q J Med* 1993; **86**: 583–593.

3. Ockene IS, Shay MJ, Alpert JS *et al.* Unexplained chest pain in patients with normal coronary arteriograms: a follow-up study of functional status. *N Engl J Med* 1980; **303**: 1249–1252.

4. de Caestecker JS, Bruce GM, Heading RC. Follow-up of patients with chest pain and normal coronary angiography: the impact of oesophageal investigations. *Eur J Gastroenterol Hepatol* 1991; **3**: 899–905.

5. Richter JE. The esophagus and noncardiac chest pain. In: Castell DO, ed. *The Esophagus*. 2nd ed. Boston, MA: Little, Brown, 1995: pp 699–724.

6. Mehta AJ, de Caestecker JS, Camm AJ, Northfield TC. Gastro-oesophageal reflux in patients with coronary artery disease: how common is it and does it matter? *Eur J Gastroenterol Hepatol* 1996; **8**: 973–978.

7. Schofield PM, Bennett DH, Whorwell PJ *et al.* Exertional gastro-oesophageal reflux: a mechanism for symptoms in patients with angina pectoris and normal coronary angiograms. *Br Med J* 1987; **294**: 1459–1461.

8. Cooke RA, Anggiansah A, Smeeton NC *et al.* Gastro-oesophageal reflux in patients with angiographically normal coronary arteries: an uncommon cause of exertional chest pain. *Br Heart J* 1994; **72**: 231–236.

9. Voskuil J-H, Cramer MJ, Breumelhof R *et al.* Prevalence of esophageal disorders in patients with chest pain newly referred to the cardiologist. *Chest* 1996; **109**: 1210–1214.

10. Smout AJPM, De Vore MS, Dalton CB, Castell DO. Cerebral potential evoked by oesophageal distension in patients with non-cardiac chest pain. *Gut* 1992; **33**: 298–302.

11. Kaski JC. Mechanisms of coronary artery spasm. *Trends Cardiovasc Med* 1991; **7**: 289–294.

12. Kemp HG. Left ventricular function in patients with the anginal syndrome and normal coronary arteriograms. *Am J Cardiol* 1973; **32**: 375–376.

13. Kaski JC. Syndrome X: a heterogeneous syndrome. Historical background, clinical presentation, electrocardiographic features, and rational patient management. An overview. In: Kaski JC, ed. *Angina Pectoris with Normal Coronary Arteries*: Syndrome X. Dordrecht: Kluwer, 1994: pp 1–18.

14. Poole-Wilson PA. Syndrome X: a non-ischaemic syndrome? – 'false positive' ST-segment shifts, ischaemia, myocardial perfusion abnor-

malities and increased sensitivity to pain in syndrome X. In: Kaski JC, ed. *Angina Pectoris with Normal Coronary Arteries: Syndrome X.* Dordrecht: Kluwer, 1994: pp 111–123.

15. Egashira K, Inou T, Hirooka Y *et al.* Evidence of impaired endothelium-dependent coronary vasal dilatation in patients with angina pectoris and normal coronary angiograms. *N Engl J Med* 1993; **328**: 1659–1664.

16. Goodfellow J, Ramsey MW, Luddington LA *et al.* Systemic endothelial dysfunction in patients with syndrome X. *Circulation* 1994; **90**(Suppl 1): 573.

17. Shapiro LM, Crake T, Poole-Wilson PA. Is altered cardiac sensation responsible for chest pain in patients with normal coronary arteries? Clinical observations during cardiac catheterisation. *Br Med J* 1988; **296**: 170–171.

18. Cannon RO, Quyyumi AA, Schenke WH *et al.* Abnormal cardiac sensitivity in patients with chest pain and normal coronary arteries. *J Am Coll Cardiol* 1990; **16**: 1359–1366.

19. Lagerqvist B, Sylven C, Waldenstrom A. Lower threshold for adenosine-induced chest pain in patients with angina and normal coronary angiograms. *Br Heart J* 1992; **68**: 282–285.

20. Rosen SD, Uren NG, Kaski JC *et al.* Coronary vasal dilator reserve, pain perception, and sex in patients with syndrome X. *Circulation* 1994; **90**: 50–60.

21. MacKenzie J, Belch J, Land D *et al.* Oesophageal ischaemia in motility disorders associated with chest pain. *Lancet* 1988; **ii**: 592–595.

22. Ghillebert G, Janssens J. Provocation tests versus 24-h pH and pressure measurements. *Eur J Gastroenterol Hepatol* 1995; **7**: 1141–1146.

23. Swarbrick ET, Hegarty JE, Bat L *et al.* Site of pain from the irritable bowel syndrome. *Lancet* 1980; **ii**: 443–446.

24. deMeester TR, O'Sullivan GC, Bermudez G *et al.* Esophageal function in patients with angina-type chest pain and normal coronary angiograms. *Ann Surg* 1982; **196**: 488–498.

25. de Caestecker JS, Blackwell JN, Brown J, Heading RC. The oesophagus as a cause of recurrent chest pain: which patient should be investigated and which tests should be used? *Lancet* 1985; **ii**: 1143–1146.

26. Hewson EG, Sinclair JW, Dalton CB, Richter JE. 24-hour esophageal pH monitoring: the most useful test for evaluating noncardiac chest pain. *Am J Med* 1991; **90**: 576–583.

27. Lam HGT, Dekker W, Kan G, Smout AJPM. Acute non-cardiac chest pain in a coronary care unit: evaluation by 24-hour pressure and pH recording of the esophagus. *Gastroenterology* 1992; **102**: 453–460.

28. Clouse RE, Carney RM. The psychological profile of non-cardiac chest

pain patients. *Eur J Gastroenterol Hepatol* 1995; **7**: 1160–1165.

29. Bass C, Wade C. Chest pain with normal coronary arteries: a comparative study of psychiatric and social morbidity. *Psychol Med* 1984; **14**: 51–61.

30. Bass C, Chambers JB, Kiff P *et al*. Panic anxiety and hyperventilation in patients with chest pain: a controlled study. *Q J Med* 1988; **69**: 949–959.

31. Richter JE, Bradley LC. Psychophysiological interactions in esophageal diseases. *Sem Gastrointest Dis* 1996; **7**: 169–184.

32. Bradley LA, Richter JE, Scarinci IC *et al*. Psychosocial and psychophysical assessment of patients with unexplained chest pain. *Am J Med* 1992; **92**(Suppl 5A): 65S-73S.

33. Scarinci IC, McDonald-Haile J, Bradley LA, Richter JE. Altered pain perception and psychosocial features among women with gastrointestinal disorders and history of abuse: a preliminary model. *Am J Med* 1994; **97**: 108–118.

34. Evans DW, Lum LC. Hyperventilation: an important cause of pseudoangina. *Lancet* 1977; **i**: 155–157.

35. Chambers JB, Kiff PJ, Gardner WN *et al*. Value of measuring end tidal partial pressure of carbon dioxide as an adjunct to treadmill exercise testing. *Br Med J* 1998; **296**: 1281–1285.

36. Cannon RO, Quyyumi AA, Mincemoyer R *et al*. Imipramine in patients with chest pain despite normal coronary angiograms. *N Engl J Med* 1994; **330**: 1411–1417.

37. Achem SR, Kolts BE, Richter JE *et al*. Treatment of acid related noncardiac chest pain: a double-blind, placebo controlled trial of omeprazole vs placebo. *Gastroenterology* 1993; **104**: A29.

38. Klimes I, Mayou RA, Pearce MJ *et al*. Psychological treatment for atypical non-cardiac chest pain: a controlled evaluation. *Psychol Med* 1990; **20**: 605–611.

39. Mayou RA, Bryant BM, Sanders D *et al*. A controlled trial of cognitive behavioural therapy for non-cardiac chest pain. *Psychol Med* 1997; **27**: 1021–1031.

40. Sanders D, Bass C, Mayou RA *et al*. Non-cardiac chest pain: why was a brief intervention apparently ineffective? *Psychol Med* 1997; **27**: 1033–1040.

11

Oesophageal infections

Oesophageal infection by *Candida* or herpes simplex may occur in otherwise healthy individuals, but is more often found in association with immunodeficiency. *Candida* oesophagitis may also occur in the elderly, following antibiotic therapy, in systemic sclerosis and in association with hypochlorhydria (either pharmacologically or surgically induced) [1]. Infection with cytomegalovirus, tuberculosis and other bacteria occur almost exclusively in the immunocompromised. Most of these infections occur in the setting of AIDS, solid organ or bone marrow transplantation, and anti-cancer and immunosuppressive therapy, including corticosteroids. Underlying malignancy, alcoholism and diabetes may also predispose to oesophageal infections. Patients with HIV infection may also present with oesophageal ulceration of uncertain cause. Oesophageal disease is common in AIDS and carries a poor prognosis, with a mean survival of less than 6 months [2]. Multiple infections may occur simultaneously in individual patients.

The overall clinical responsibility for patients with any of the conditions listed above is not usually with the gastroenterologist. His/her role will largely be subsidiary, in particular in helping the referring physician with diagnosis. This chapter will therefore emphasize clinical presentation and the role of endoscopy. The latter is usually the investigation of choice, the abnormalities demonstrated by a barium swallow not being sufficiently specific to be routinely useful diagnostically [3]. Treatment regimes will only be discussed briefly; for more detailed accounts of the latter the reader is referred to several excellent recent reviews [1,3–5].

The commonest symptoms of infectious oesophagitis are dysphagia, odynophagia (painful swallowing) and retrosternal pain. Systemic symptoms and symptoms in other organs depend on the underlying infection (Table 11.1). Complications of oesophageal ulceration, including haemorrhage, perforation and fistulation may also occur.

Table 11.1 Summary of presenting symptoms (%) in patients with oesophageal infection (based on reference 1, comprising 416 patients from 57 published studies, with permission of the publisher)

	Candida	CMV	HSV	TB	HIV ulcer
Dysphagia and/or odynophagia	63	59	79	64	95
Oral lesions	37	0	29	6	27
Nausea/vomiting	5	42	15	1	2
Abdominal pain	5	19	2	2	5
Weight loss	1	25	2	35	27
Fever	2	20	4	20	12
Asymptomatic	23	0	0	0	0

CMV = cytomegalovirus; HSV = herpes simplex virus; TB = tuberculosis; HIV = human immunodeficiency virus.

CANDIDA

Candida oesophagitis is sometimes asymptomatic, but two-thirds complain of dysphagia and/or odynophagia. Only one-third will have associated oral *Candida*. Systemic symptoms are unusual (Table 11.1). It is often the first manifestation of AIDS.

The endoscopic appearance ranges from a few, tiny, raised white plaques through to large, confluent, linear nodular plaques with ulceration [6]. Mucosal plaques may also occur with the other oesophageal infections listed below. Small 'plaques' may be due to swallowed food debris, but those due to *Candida* cannot be washed off and usually bleed when brushed away.

The diagnosis of *Candida* can easily be confirmed by appropriate staining of biopsy specimens. For patients with AIDS who present with oesophageal symptoms the most likely diagnosis is *Candida*, especially if oral lesions are present. It may be cost-effective to treat these patients blindly and reserve endoscopy for those who do not respond [3].

The infection can usually be treated with topical clotrimazole (10 mg troches, five times daily for 5–10 days) if the underlying immune problem is minimal. For those with more severe problems systemic oral fluconazole, (100–200 mg daily for 1–2 weeks) is the treatment of choice. If there is granulocytopenia (e.g. following bone marrow transplantation, chemotherapy or in advanced AIDS) intravenous amphotericin may be necessary.

Although the majority of patients with AIDS respond to oral fluconazole, most will relapse within 3 months [7]. Prophylactic treatment may therefore be required, but its value has to be weighed against the risk of emergence of fluconazole-resistant strains.

CYTOMEGALOVIRUS (CMV)

The majority of the world's population has been infected with CMV and the DNA can be found in most organs [8]. Reactivation of the virus may occur in the immunocompromised. CMV oesophagitis is particularly common in transplantation patients and in AIDS if the CD4 lymphocyte count is less than $100/mm^3$. The onset of symptoms is usually more gradual and more generalized than with *Candida*. Two-thirds complain of dysphagia and/or odynophagia, oral lesions do not occur, but more generalized symptoms of nausea, vomiting, weight-loss, fever and diarrhoea are common (Table 11.1).

Serological tests are unhelpful, with too many false-positive and false-negative results [1]. Endoscopy will reveal lesions in the mid and distal oesophagus. Characteristically, superficial serpiginous ulcers are seen that vary in size from 1 mm to 2 cm in length. Deep ulcers are unusual [9]. Biopsies should be taken, particularly from the ulcer base to sample infected fibroblasts and endothelial cells [10]. The histological features include large cells in the subepithelial layer with intranuclear inclusions, a halo around the nucleus and multiple small cytoplasmic inclusions.

Treatment is by ganciclovir (5 mg/kg 12-hourly i.v. for 2 weeks) or foscarnet (60 mg/kg 8-hourly i.v. for 2 weeks), but relapses are common. Maintenance therapy is therefore sometimes necessary. Prophylactic treatment is often recommended when immunodeficiency is severe [4].

HERPES SIMPLEX VIRUS (HSV)

Most patients with HSV oesophagitis present acutely with dysphagia and/or odynophagia, one-third also having oral lesions. Systemic upsets are unusual (Table 11.1). In the immunocompetent host the infection is usually short-lived and does not require treatment, but it may be severe and prolonged in patients with immunodeficiency. For the latter group complications include strictures, oesophago-respiratory fistulae, HSV pneumonia and disseminated infection. It is uncommon in AIDS until the CD4 lymphocyte count is less than $100/mm^3$.

At endoscopy the appearance ranges from small vesicles through small, clearly defined ulcers with slightly raised edges, to longer ulcers with inflammatory exudate. In severe cases the whole oesophagus may be involved [11,12]. The diagnosis can be made by histology of biopsies from the squamous epithelium at the margins of the ulcer. The characteristic findings include multinucleate giant cells and intranuclear inclusions. Culture of the ulcer edge is also helpful [12].

Acyclovir (200–400 mg five times daily orally, or $250 \, mg/m^2$ 8-hourly i.v. for 2 weeks), or foscarnet (60 mg/kg 8-hourly i.v. for 2 weeks) for resistant strains, are the treatments of choice. These drugs suppress but do not eradicate the infection. Maintenance treatment may therefore have to be given.

MYCOBACTERIA

Oesophagitis due to *Mycobacterium tuberculosis* usually presents with dysphagia and/or odynophagia, together with pulmonary symptoms, fever and weight loss (Table 11.1). Infected mediastinal nodes may perforate into the oesophagus. Oesophago-respiratory fistulae may occur. Infection with *M. avium intracellulare*, though relatively common in AIDS patients, rarely affects the oesophagus.

The endoscopic findings include shallow ulcers ranging in size from minute to large [13,14]. Occasionally, the mucosa may be heaped up and resemble a carcinoma [14,15]. The diagnosis can be confirmed from appropriately stained or cultured biopsy material.

Standard antituberculous therapy is usually effective, but surgery may be required for mechanical complications. *M. avium intracellulare* is much less responsive to treatment [1].

OTHER BACTERIA

Bacteria normally present in the mouth and upper respiratory tract may infect the oesophagus in granulocytopenic patients. They complain of the usual symptoms of infectious oesophagitis, dysphagia and/or odynophagia. The endoscopic findings range from oesophageal erythema to extensive ulcerative oesophagitis with exudate [1]. Diagnosis is made from Gram staining of biopsy specimens. Treatment is with the appropriate antibiotic.

HIV-ASSOCIATED OESOPHAGEAL ULCER OF UNCERTAIN CAUSE

Oesophageal ulcers of uncertain cause may accompany HIV infection. Dysphagia and/or odynophagia are almost invariable and oral lesions are common. They may occur at the time of seroconversion (usually 2–3 weeks after exposure to the virus), when it is associated with a flu-like illness of approximately 2 weeks duration, or much later when the CD4 lymphocyte count falls below $50/\text{mm}^3$ [1,4].

The diagnosis is made by endoscopy. The appearance ranges from small superficial aphthoid lesions to large ulcers. Infectious causes must be excluded by biopsy of the ulcer edges and base.

Once infection has been excluded prednisolone should be administered, initially 40 mg/d [4]. Most patients rapidly improve. However, corticosteroids can expose the patient to the risk of the other oesophageal infections listed above.

REFERENCES

1. Baehr PH, McDonald GB. Esophageal infections: risk factors, presentation, diagnosis, and treatment. *Gastroenterology* 1994; **106**: 509–532.
2. Connolly GM, Hawkins D, Harcourt-Webster JN *et al.* Oesophageal symptoms, their causes, treatment, and prognosis in patients with the acquired immunodeficiency syndrome. *Gut* 1989; **30**: 1033–1039.
3. Dieterich DT, Wilcox CM. Diagnosis and treatment of esophageal diseases associated with HIV infection. *Am J Gastroenterol* 1996; **91**: 2265–2269.
4. Wilcox CM, Mönkemüller KE. Review article: The therapy of gastrointestinal infections associated with the acquired immunodeficiency syndrome. *Aliment Pharmacol Ther* 1997; **11**: 425–443.
5. Noyer CM, Simon D. Oral and esophageal disorders. *Gastroenterol Clin North Am* 1997; **26**: 241–257.
6. Kodsi BE, Wickremesinghe PC, Kozinn PJ *et al. Candida* esophagitis. A prospective study of 27 cases. *Gastroenterology* 1976; **71**: 715–719.
7. Laine L. The natural history of esophageal candidiasis after successful treatment in patients with AIDS. *Gastroenterology* 1994; **107**: 744–746.
8. Myerson D, Hackman RC, Nelson JA *et al.* Widespread presence of histologically occult cytomegalovirus. *Hum Pathol* 1984; **15**: 430–439.
9. Wilcox CM, Straub RF, Schwartz DA. Prospective endoscopic characterisation of cytomegalovirus esophagitis in AIDS. *Gastrointest Endosc* 1994; **40**: 481–484.
10. McDonald GB, Sharma P, Hackman *et al.* Esophageal infections in immunosuppressed patients after marrow transplantation. *Gastroenterology* 1984; **88**: 1111–1117.
11. Byard RW, Champion MC, Orizaga M. Variability in the clinical presentation and endoscopic findings of herpetic esophagitis. *Endoscopy* 1987; **19**: 153–155.
12. McBane RD, Gross JB. Herpes esophagitis: clinical syndrome, endoscopic appearance, and diagnosis in 23 patients. *Gastrointest Endosc* 1991; **37**: 600–603.
13. Dow C. Oesophageal tuberculosis: four cases. *Gut* 1981; **22**: 234–236.
14. Pina Cabral JE, Toste M, Correia Leitao M *et al.* Endoscopic diagnosis of esophageal tuberculosis. *Am J Gastroenterol* 1990; **85**: 1431–1432.
15. Wort SJ, Puleston JM, Hill PD, Holdstock GE. Primary tuberculosis of the oesophagus. *Lancet* 1997; **349**: 1072.

12

Tumours

MALIGNANT TUMOURS

The majority of malignant tumours of the oesophagus are squamous cell carcinoma or adenocarcinoma. Until recently squamous cell carcinoma was the most common in the Western world, with a reported incidence of approximately 6/100 000/year [1]. This compares with an incidence of up to 165/100 000/year in patients in parts of China and Iran. The incidence rises with age. The cause is unknown, but risk factors include poverty, poor nutrition, alcoholism, tobacco, human papilloma virus in a small number of cases, caustic strictures, postcricoid web and achalasia. The most common site is the mid-oesophagus, but it may occur proximally or distally.

Adenocarcinoma of the oesophagus has been reported to be increasing in incidence more rapidly than any other malignancy in the Western world and is now of similar incidence to squamous cell carcinoma (Chapter 6). It affects the mid- and lower thirds of the oesophagus. Most cases, together with many cases of adenocarcinoma of the cardia, arise from Barrett's metaplasia, a consequence of gastro-oesophageal reflux.

Rare malignant tumours of the oesophagus include oat cell carcinoma, malignant melanoma, carcinosarcoma [1] and lymphoma [2]. Lymphoma and Kaposi's sarcoma may occur in AIDS [3].

The clinical features, prognosis, assessment and treatment are similar for squamous cell carcinoma and adenocarcinoma and will therefore be considered together.

Clinical features

Squamous cell carcinoma and adenocarcinoma of the oesophagus have a poor prognosis, with few patients surviving more than 5 years. The tumours spread locally, by lymphatics and by blood.

The most common presenting symptom is progressive dysphagia, often initially to solids, but later to solids and liquids. Swallowing may be painful. Regurgitation, aspiration, hoarseness, anorexia, weight loss and haematemesis are common. There may be symptoms due to local spread, particularly development of an oesophago-respiratory fistula.

Investigations

Macroscopically the tumour may be nothing more than a discoloured patch in the oesophageal mucosa, an ulcer, or a fungating or stenosing lesion. By the time dysphagia is present the lesion will usually be detectable by barium swallow, but a double-contrast technique may reveal earlier lesions. Characteristically the appearances are of an irregular filling defect or long stricture (Figure 12.1). There may be distortion of the long axis of the barium column by a fixed tumour.

CT scanning is useful for assessing mediastinal spread when considering surgery, but when available endoscopic ultrasound is superior. The latter technique is the most accurate method for assessing the depth of tumour within the wall of the oesophagus and also for detecting regional node enlargement [4]. The main limitation of endoscopic ultrasound is failure of the probe to penetrate a stenosing lesion.

Endoscopy is necessary to obtain tissue for histology. Endoscopic surveillance of Barrett's oesophagus has been described elsewhere (Chapter 6). The sensitivity of endoscopy for the detection of squamous cell carcinoma may be increased by spraying the mucosa with Lugol's iodine [5].

Other investigational techniques whose role is not yet clear include nuclear magnetic resonance scanning and spiral CT.

Some surgeons will perform laparoscopy to assess resectability, particularly for low lesions [6].

Treatment

Probably the best chance of permanent cure, particularly for adenocarcinoma, is surgical resection, but the 5-year survival is only about 10% [7]. Approximately one-third of cases are resectable and the operative mortality is high [7,8]. Some recommend 'palliative' resection as the most suitable treatment for dysphagia even when distant metastases are known to be present [9].

External beam radiotherapy as the primary treatment without surgical resection, particularly for squamous cell carcinoma, has also reported 5-year survival figures of about 10% [10,11]. Although squamous cell carcinomas are sometimes considered more radiosensitive than adenocarcinoma, no difference was found in one large series [10]. A prospective

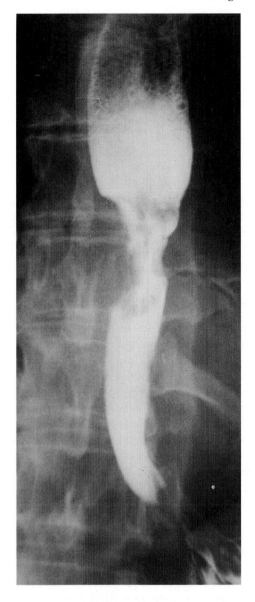

Figure 12.1 Barium swallow illustrating a large malignant tumour in the mid-oesophagus.

randomized trial of surgical resection against radiotherapy has not been completed [11].

Neither preoperative nor postoperative external beam radiotherapy [12–14] nor adjuvant chemotherapy [15–17] has improved outcome following surgery. However, a recent trial of fluorouracil and cis-platinum together with external beam radiotherapy improved the 3-year survival following surgery for adenocarcinoma to 32%, compared with 6% for those undergoing surgery alone [18].

Early carcinoma

There are now reports of successful eradication of early carcinoma of the oesophagus by endoscopic resection [19] or photodynamic therapy [20–22]. In one of these series a 75% 5-year disease-specific survival was reported for 123 patients with T1 or T2 squamous cell carcinoma or adenocarcinoma [22].

Palliative treatment

In practice the aim of treatment for most patients with carcinoma of the oesophagus is palliation. They have a very limited life expectancy and every attempt should be made to improve swallowing, maintain nutrition, control pain and minimize time spent in hospital.

External beam radiotherapy will improve dysphagia in most patients depending on tumour size [11]. Radiotherapy can also be given intra-luminally ('brachytherapy') [23]. Neither type of radiotherapy should be given in the presence of an oesophago-respiratory fistula [24].

Other means of improving swallowing include simple oesophageal dilatation, intubation, thermal laser treatment and ethanol injection.

Simple dilatation of tumours with a suitable bougie is moderately effective but associated with rapid recurrence of dysphagia [25].

Intubation is the most widely used palliative treatment. Various semi-rigid stents are available (Atkinson, Wilson–Cook). These have flanges to help prevent slipping. The intubation can be carried out under benzodiazepine sedation, preferably with X-ray control [26]. A 9% perforation rate has been reported [27]. It may be technically impossible to pass a tube through a sharply angulated tumour and the technique is unsuitable for high oesophageal tumours. Other problems include bolus obstruction and tumour occlusion by growth into the lumen. More recently expanding metal mesh stents have become available. These are undoubtedly simpler and safer to insert, and are associated with easier swallowing, but are substantially more expensive [28]. A fistula into the respiratory tract can often be occluded by a stent, sometimes wrapped in an expandable polyurethane sponge [26].

Thermal ablation, particularly using the Nd–YAG laser, is now an established palliative treatment for exophytic tumours [29]. Unfortunately, rapid regrowth necessitates repeat procedures, but the interval between treatment sessions can be substantially increased by adjuvant luminal [30] or external beam radiotherapy [31].

Randomized controlled trials comparing intubation and laser ablation have failed to show any consistent overall superiority for either treatment [32,33].

Ethanol-induced necrosis of exophytic tumours is also becoming established as a relatively simple, safe and cheap form of treatment [34]. Small amounts (0.5–1 ml) of absolute ethanol are injected into the tumour at multiple sites commencing distally. If necessary the lumen is first dilated to 12 mm. If the tumour occludes the lumen ethanol is injected proximally and the procedure is repeated in 3–7 days. Re-injections are needed approximately monthly.

BENIGN TUMOURS

Benign tumours of the oesophagus are rare and often asymptomatic.

Leiomyoma

This is the most common benign tumour, but much less common than in the stomach [35,36]. They usually occur intramurally and may grow into the mediastinum. If symptoms occur these include dysphagia or the effects of a tumour mass in the mediastinum. They may ulcerate and bleed.

Benign polyps

Benign polyps are the second most common benign tumour and may consist of fatty, fibrous, muscular or inflammatory tissue [35]. They may present with haemorrhage and can sometimes be removed endoscopically.

Granular cell tumour

These are probably derived from Schwann cells [37] and are often multiple and often asymptomatic [38].

Pseudotumour

Lesions resembling exophytic tumours have been described as a consequence of gastro-oesophageal reflux [39] and tuberculosis [40].

REFERENCES

1. Mannell A. Tumours. In: Bouchier IAD, Allan RN, Hodgson HJF, Keighley MRB, eds. *Gastroenterology – Clinical Science and Practice*. 2nd ed. Philadelphia, PA: WB Saunders, 1993: pp 119–166.
2. Taal BG, Van Heerde P, Somers R. Isolated primary oesophageal involvement by lymphoma: a rare cause of dysphagia: two case histories and a review of other published data. *Gut* 1993; **34**: 994–998.
3. Dieterich DT, Wilcox CM. Diagnosis and treatment of esophageal diseases associated with HIV infection. *Am J Gastroenterol* 1996; **91**: 2265–2269.
4. Fockens P, van Lanschot JJB, Tytgat GN. The role of endosonography in esophageal carcinoma: who should get it, who should do it? *Scand J Gastroenterol* 1996; **31**(Suppl 218): 82–85.
5. Yokoyama A, Ohmori T, Makuuchi H *et al.* Successful screening for early esophageal cancer in alcoholics using endoscopy and mucosa iodine staining. *Cancer* 1995; **76**: 928–934.
6. Molloy RC, McCourtney JS, Anderson JR. Laparoscopy in the management of patients with cancer of the gastric cardia and oesophagus. *Br J Surg* 1995; **82**: 352–354.
7. Sagar PM, Gauperaa T, Sue Ling H *et al.* An audit of the treatment of cancer of the oesophagus. *Gut* 1994; **35**: 941–945.
8. Oliver SE, Robertson CS, Logan RFA. Oesophageal cancer: a population-based study of survival after treatment. *Br J Surg* 1992; **79**: 1321–1325.
9. Ellis FH. Surgical palliation: esophageal resection – a surgeon's opinion. In: Delaru NC, Wilkins EW, Wong J, eds. *International Trends in Thoracic Surgery*, vol 4. St Louis, MO: CV Mosby, 1988: pp 375–381.
10. Slevin NJ, Stout R. Carcinoma of the oesophagus – a review of 108 cases treated by radiotherapy. *Clin Radiol* 1989; **40**: 200–203.
11. Earlam RJ, Johnson L. 101 oesophageal cancers: a surgeon uses radiotherapy. *Ann R Coll Surg Engl* 1990; **72**: 32–40.
12. Naunheim KS, Petruska PJ, Roy TS *et al.* Preoperative chemotherapy and radiotherapy for esophageal carcinoma. *J Thorac Cardiovasc Surg* 1992; **5**: 887–893.
13. Launois B, Delarue D, Campion JP, Karbaol M. Preoperative radiotherapy for carcinoma of the esophagus. *Surg Gynecol Obstet* 1981; **153**: 690–692.
14. Tenière P, Hay JM, Fingerhut A, Fagniez PL. Postoperative radiation therapy does not increase survival after curative resection for squamous cell carcinoma of the middle and lower esophagus as

shown by a multicentre controlled trial. *Surg Gynecol Obstet* 1991; **173**: 123–130.

15. Schlag PM. Randomised trial of preoperative chemotherapy for squamous cell cancer of the esophagus. *Arch Surg* 1992; **127**: 1446–1450.

16. Japanese Esophageal Oncology Group. A comparison of chemotherapy and radiotherapy as adjuvant treatment to surgery for esophageal carcinoma. *Chest* 1993; **104**: 203–207.

17. Apinop C, Puttisak P, Preecha N. A prospective study of combined therapy in esophageal cancer. *Hepatogastroenterology* 1994; **41**: 391–393.

18. Walsh TN, Noonan N, Hollywood D *et al.* A comparison of multimodal therapy and surgery for esophageal adenocarcinoma. *N Engl J Med* 1996; **335**: 462–467.

19. Takeshita K, Tani M, Inoue H *et al.* Endoscopic treatment of early oesophageal or gastric cancer. *Gut* 1997; **40**: 123–127.

20. Overholt B, Panjehpour M, Tefftellar E, Rose M. Photodynamic therapy for treatment of early adenocarcinoma in Barrett's esophagus. *Gastrointest Endosc* 1993; **39**: 73–76.

21. Regula J, MacRobert AJ, Gorchein A *et al.* Photosensitisation and photodynamic therapy of oesophageal, duodenal, and colorectal tumours using 5 aminolaevulinic acid induced protoporphyrin IX – a pilot study. *Gut* 1995; **36**: 67–75.

22. Sibille A, Lambert R, Souquet JC *et al.* Long term survival after photodynamic therapy for esophageal cancer. *Gastroenterology* 1995; **108**: 337–344.

23. Rowland CG, Pagliero KM. Intracavitary irradiation for oesophageal malignancy. In: Bennett JR, Hunt RH, eds. *Therapeutic Endoscopy and Radiology of the Gut*. 2nd ed. London: Chapman & Hall, 1990: pp 77–81.

24. Dakkak M, Bennett JR. Palliation of oesophageal cancer. In: Farthing MJG, ed. *Clinical Challenges in Gastroenterology*. London: Dunitz, 1996: pp 1–13.

25. Heit HA, Johnson LF, Siegel SR, Boyce HW. Palliative dilatation for dysphagia in esophageal carcinoma. *Ann Intern Med* 1978; **89**: 629–631.

26. Atkinson M. Endoscopic intubation of oesophageal malignant obstruction. In: Bennett JR, Hunt RH, eds. *Therapeutic Endoscopy and Radiology of the Gut*. 2nd ed. London: Chapman & Hall, 1990: pp 53–64.

27. Bennett JR. Intubation of gastro-oesophageal malignancies: a survey of current practice in Britain. *Gut* 1981; **22**: 336–338.

28. Sturgess RP, Morris AI. Metal stents in the oesophagus. *Gut* 1995; **37**: 593–594.

29. Bown SG. Laser disobliteration for advanced gastrointestinal malignancy. In: Bennett JR, Hunt RH, eds. *Therapeutic Endoscopy and Radiology of the Gut.* 2nd ed. London: Chapman & Hall, 1990: pp 65–76.

30. Shmueli E, Srivastava E, Dawes PJDK *et al.* Combination of laser treatment and intraluminal radiotherapy for malignant dysphagia. *Gut* 1996; **38**: 803–805.

31. Sargeant IR, Tobias JS, Blackman G *et al.* Radiotherapy enhances laser palliation of malignant dysphagia: a randomised study. *Gut* 1997; **40**: 362–369.

32. Alderson D, Wright PD. Laser recanalisation versus endoscopic intubation in the palliation of malignant dysphasia. *Br J Surg* 1990; **77**: 1151–1153.

33. Adam A, Ellul J, Watkinson AF *et al.* Palliation of inoperable esophageal carcinoma: a prospective randomized trial of laser therapy and stent placement. *Radiology* 1997; **202**: 344–348.

34. Nwokolo CU, Payne-James JJ, Silk DBA *et al.* Palliation of malignant dysphagia by ethanol induced tumour necrosis. *Gut* 1994; **35**: 299–303.

35. Plachta A, Benign tumors of the esophagus. Review of literature and report of 99 cases. *Am J Gastroenterol* 1962; **38**: 639–652.

36. Seremetis MG, Lyons WS, de Guzmann VC, Peabody JW. Leiomyomata of the esophagus. *Cancer* 1976; **38**: 2166–2177.

37. Fisher ER, Wechsler H. Granular cell myoblastoma – a misnomer. Electron microscopic and histochemical evidence concerning its Schwann cell derivation and nature (granular cell Schwannoma). *Cancer* 1962; **15**: 936–954.

38. Goldblum JR, Rice TW, Zuccaro G, Richter JE. Granular cell tumours of the esophagus: a clinical and pathologic study of 13 cases. *Ann Thorac Surg* 1996; **62**: 860–865.

39. Staples DC, Knodell RG, Johnson LF. Inflammatory pseudotumor of the esophagus. A complication of gastroesophageal reflux. *Gastrointest Endosc* 1978; **24**: 175–176.

40. Wort SJ, Puleston JM, Hill PD, Holdstock GE. Primary tuberculosis of the oesophagus. *Lancet* 1997; **349**: 1072.

13

The oesophagus in systemic and cutaneous diseases

SYSTEMIC SCLEROSIS

At least two-thirds of patients with systemic sclerosis (scleroderma) have oesophageal involvement, this being the most commonly affected part of the alimentary tract [1]. The condition affects the smooth muscle, i.e. mid and lower oesophagus. Pathologically the changes are of smooth muscle atrophy, arteriolar sclerosis and collagen deposition [2].

The commonest symptoms are gastro-oesophageal reflux and dysphagia. The latter is usually due to distal oesophageal dysmotility/amotility, but can be due to oesophagitis, peptic stricture, or a carcinoma superimposed on columnar (Barrett's) metaplasia. A benign stricture may occur in up to 42% of patients and columnar metaplasia in up to 37% [3]. The oesophageal symptoms may be the first presentation of systemic sclerosis [4].

Radiology, endoscopy, manometry and pH monitoring may all be helpful diagnostically. A plain chest X-ray may reveal an air-filled atonic oesophagus with a fluid level. Contrast radiology will reveal poor or absent distal peristalsis and a patulous oesophagogastric sphincter with free reflux. It may also reveal a stricture. Endoscopy is essential to assess the severity of reflux-induced mucosal damage and columnar metaplasia. Stationary manometry is the most specific diagnostic test, the changes including a hypotensive lower oesophageal sphincter and absence of distal peristalsis, proximal peristalsis being maintained [5]. The severity and duration of oesophageal acid exposure can only be assessed by pH monitoring.

The changes in oesophageal function are not necessarily rapidly progressive in that no alteration was observed in 16/17 patients restudied after a mean period of $3\frac{1}{2}$ years [5].

There is no satisfactory treatment for the underlying disease process.

Motility enhancing drugs are of minimal, if any, benefit [3]. Omeprazole is immensely beneficial as treatment for the gastro-oesophageal reflux [6,7], but high doses may be required.

Surgical treatment of reflux is often not satisfactory. In view of the poor or absent oesophageal peristalsis a standard fundoplication may exacerbate dysphagia. Because there is often associated oesophageal shortening, a combined gastroplasty/fundoplication has been reported to be successful [8,9]. Others suggest oesophageal replacement [10].

MIXED CONNECTIVE TISSUE DISEASE

This is a condition with features of systemic sclerosis, systemic lupus erythematosus and polymyositis. The oesophageal changes are similar to those of systemic sclerosis [11].

POLYMYOSITIS AND DERMATOMYOSITIS

As well as involving the smooth muscle segment of the oesophagus, polymyositis and dermatomyositis may also affect the striated (proximal) segment [12]. This will manifest as oropharyngeal dysphagia with frequent aspiration and nasal regurgitation. Treatment is that of the underlying myositis.

OTHER CONNECTIVE TISSUE DISEASES

Impaired peristalsis and lower oesophageal sphincter hypotonia have been described in systemic lupus erythematosus, rheumatoid arthritis and Sjögren's syndrome [3], but severe oesophageal symptoms are unusual.

CHRONIC IDIOPATHIC PSEUDO-OBSTRUCTION

Oesophageal involvement in chronic idiopathic pseudo-obstruction is common and mimics achalasia, with reduced or absent peristalsis and incomplete lower oesophageal sphincter relaxation [13]. However, dysphagia is unusual [14].

DIABETES MELLITUS, ALCOHOL, AMYLOID

Oesophageal motility disorders have been described in all of these conditions, but are rarely clinically relevant [3].

BULLOUS CUTANEOUS CONDITIONS

Diagnosis of bullous cutaneous conditions is usually straightforward clinically, but can be confirmed by specific histological features in skin or mucosal biopsies.

Epidermolysis bullosa

There are several types of epidermolysis bullosa, all characterized by mucocutaneous blistering. They are classified according to the histological level of blister formation [15]. Clinical oesophageal involvement with dysphagia occurs particularly in the dystrophic forms – approximately three-quarters in the recessive type and one-fifth in the dominant. It is much less common in the junctional and simplex forms [16]. Minimal trauma to the skin and mucous membranes may give rise to bulla formation followed by scarring. The whole of the oesophagus may be affected, with multiple webs and strictures. Skin manifestations are usually striking. Steroids and phenytoin have been reported to be beneficial as has careful stricture dilatation, but some patients require oesophageal resection [17].

Bullous pemphigoid and cicatricial pemphigoid

Bullous pemphigoid is a chronic blistering condition affecting the elderly. Oesophageal involvement is rare, but when present may manifest itself by dysphagia, bleeding, and sloughing of the epithelium as a cast [18,19].

Cicatricial pemphigoid affects the mucous membranes of the mouth, eyes and genitalia. It is complicated by scarring. Oesophageal involvement may result in webs and strictures, which may require dilatation [20,21].

Each of these conditions usually responds to prednisolone, commencing with a dose of 80 mg daily.

Pemphigus vulgaris

Pemphigus vulgaris is a condition of the skin and oral mucosa affecting younger adults and characterized by more flaccid bullae. Oesophageal involvement is rare, but when present manifests itself similarly to bullous pemphigoid [22].

STEVENS–JOHNSON SYNDROME

This condition can rarely affect the oesophagus, with blistering and desquamation, followed by stricture formation [23].

LICHEN PLANUS

Lichen planus is a common skin condition that often affects the oesophagus, but usually without symptoms [24]. In more severe cases there may be painful dysphagia, which often responds to corticosteroids [25].

BEHÇET'S SYNDROME

Oesophageal ulceration in Behçet's syndrome is rare [26].

REFERENCES

1. Poirier TJ, Rankin GB. Gastrointestinal manifestations of progressive systemic scleroderma based on a review of 364 cases. *Am J Gastroenterol* 1972; **58**: 30–44.
2. Treacy WL, Baggenstoss AH, Slocum BCH *et al.* Scleroderma of the esophagus. A correlation of histologic and physiologic findings. *Ann Intern Med* 1963; **59**: 351–356.
3. Yarze JC. Esophageal manifestations in systemic diseases. In: Castell DO, ed. *The Esophagus*. 2nd ed. Boston, MA: Little, Brown, 1995: pp 361–378.
4. Kinder RR, Fleischmann R. Systemic scleroderma: a review of organ systems. *Int J Dermatol* 1974; **13**: 362–395.
5. Dantas RO, Meneghelli UG, Oliveira RB, Villanova MG. Esophageal dysfunction does not always worsen in systemic sclerosis. *J Clin Gastroenterol* 1993; **17**: 281–285.
6. Hendel L, Hage E, Hendel J, Stentof T. Omeprazole in long-term treatment of severe gastro-oesophageal reflux disease in patients with systemic sclerosis. *Aliment Pharmacol Ther* 1992; **6**: 565–577.
7. Hendel J, Hendel L, Hage E *et al.* Monitoring of omeprazole treatment in gastro-oesophageal reflux disease. *Eur J Gastroenterol Hepatol* 1996; **8**: 417–420.
8. Orringer MB *et al.* Combined Collis gastroplasty–fundoplication operations for scleroderma reflux esophagitis. *Surgery* 1981; **90**: 624–630.
9. Pearson FG, Cooper JD, Patterson GA *et al.* Gastroplasty and fundoplication for complex reflux problems: long-term results. *Ann Surg* 1982; **206**: 473–481.
10. Mansour KA, Malone CE. Surgery for scleroderma of the esophagus: a 12 year experience. *Ann Thorac Surg* 1988; **46**: 513–514.
11. Marshall JB, Kretschmar JM, Gerhardt DC *et al.* Gastro-intestinal manifestations of mixed connective tissue disease. *Gastroenterology* 1990; **98**: 1232–1238.

12. Turner R, Lipshutz W, Miller W *et al.* Esophageal dysfunction in collagen disease. *Am J Med Sci* 1973; **265**: 191–199.
13. Schuffler MD, Pope CE. Esophageal motor dysfunction in idiopathic intestinal pseudoobstruction. *Gastroenterology* 1976; **70**: 677–682.
14. Schuffler MD, Rohrmann CA, Chaffe RG *et al.* Chronic intestinal pseudo-obstruction. A report of 27 cases and review of the literature. *Medicine* 1981; **60**: 173–196.
15. Fine J-D, Bauer EA, Briggaman RA *et al.* Revised clinical and laboratory criteria for sub-types of inherited epidermolysis bullosa. *J Am Acad Dermatol* 1991; **24**: 119–135.
16. Travis SPL, McGrath JA, Turnbull AJ *et al.* Oral and gastrointestinal manifestations of epidermolysis bullosa. *Lancet* 1992; **340**: 1505–1506.
17. Touloukian RJ, Schonholz SM, Gryboski JD *et al.* Perioperative considerations in esophageal replacement for epidermolysis bullosa: report of two cases successfully treated by colon interposition. *Am J Gastroenterol* 1988; **83**: 857–861.
18. Foroozan P, Enta T, Winship DH, Trier JS. Loss and regurgitation of the esophageal mucosa in pemphigoid. *Gastroenterology* 1967; **52**: 548–558.
19. Eng TY, Hogan WJ, Jordon RG. Oesophageal involvement in bullous pemphigoid. A possible cause of gastrointestinal haemorrhage. *Br J Dermatol* 1978; **99**: 207–210.
20. Al-Kutoubi MA, Eliot C. Oesophageal involvement in benign mucous membrane pemphigoid. *Clin Radiol* 1984; **35**: 131–135.
21. Isolauri J, Airo I. Benign mucous membrane pemphigoid involving the esophagus: a report of two cases treated with dilation. *Gastrointest Endosc* 1989; **35**: 569–571.
22. Kaneko F, Mori M, Tsukinaga I, Miura Y. Pemphigus vulgaris of esophageal mucosa. *Arch Dermatol* 1985; **121**: 272–273.
23. Stein MR, Thompson CK, Sawicki JE, Martel AJ. Esophageal stricture complicating Stevens–Johnson syndrome. A case report. *Am J Gastroenterol* 1974; **62**: 435–439.
24. Dickens CM, Heseltine D, Walton S *et al.* The oesophagus in lichen planus: an endoscopic study. *Br Med J* 1990; **300**: 84.
25. Souto P, Sofia C, Cabral JP *et al.* Oesophageal lichen planus. *Eur J Gastroenterol Hepatol* 1979; **9**: 725–727.
26. Anti M, Marra G, Rapaccini GL *et al.* Esophageal involvement in Behçet's Syndrome. *J Clin Gastroenterol* 1986; **8**: 514–519.

14

Structural abnormalities

HIATUS HERNIA

Three types of hiatus hernia are recognized: sliding, para-oesophageal (rolling), and mixed (Figure 14.1).

Sliding hiatus hernia

A sliding hiatus hernia is by far the commonest type. It can be demonstrated radiologically in well over 50% of the adult population. Although often of pathophysiological importance in gastro-oesophageal reflux (Chapter 2) the term is not synonymous with this condition. Many patients with reflux do not have a hernia and vice versa [1]. In most subjects in whom a hernia can be demonstrated it is probably of no clinical relevance at all. Certainly, patients with a hernia should not be subject to operative repair for non-specific abdominal symptoms.

Anaemia has long been recognized in association with hiatus hernia [2], but the published studies date from the 1960s, before the availability of fibreoptic oesophagogastroduodenoscopy and colonoscopy. Other causes for the anaemia in these patients may not therefore have been adequately excluded. However, superficial ulcerative lesions may occur within a large hernia sac, particularly at or near the region of the diaphragm [2–4], which could conceivably result in occult blood loss. These lesions can often be healed by acid suppression [5].

Para-oesophageal (rolling) hernia

A para-oesophageal hernia is characterized by herniation of the gastric fundus and subsequently more of the stomach, often with volvulus. Other

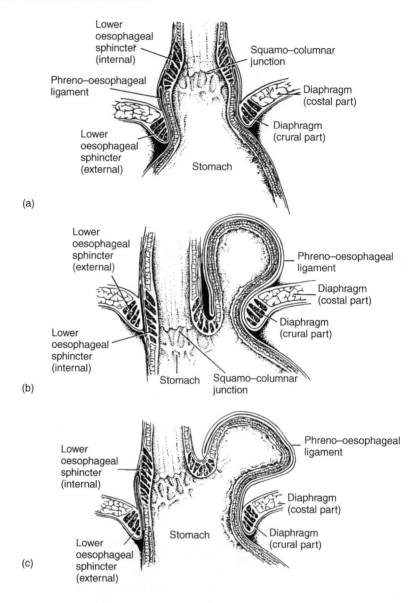

Figure 14.1 The different types of hiatus hernia: **(a)** sliding; **(b)** rolling; **(c)** mixed. Compare with the normal lower oesophageal sphincter illustrated in Figure 2.1. (Source: redrawn from Rourk RM, Mittal RK. Hiatal hernia. When is it responsible for symptoms? In: Barkin JS, Rogers AI, eds. *Difficult Decisions in Digestive Diseases*. St Louis, MO: CV Mosby, 1994: pp 43–50, with permission of the publisher.)

organs may also herniate. The cardia of the stomach remains in its normal location beneath the diaphragm.

It is a relatively rare condition, usually presenting late in life. The symptoms are often initially vague, including nausea, fullness or pain after meals and symptoms of a space-occupying lesion in the chest. Vomiting is rare.

It may present acutely with bleeding, volvulus or incarceration. The latter two are characterized by severe pain and may progress to ischaemic necrosis with perforation. The mortality is high [6,7]. It is therefore usually suggested that these hernias be repaired if discovered before major complications have developed.

Mixed hernia

A mixed hernia may present with symptoms of a para-oesophageal hernia, gastro-oesophageal reflux or a combination of these [8]. Surgical repair is usually recommended.

WEBS

Many webs are asymptomatic, but they may present with intermittent solid food dysphagia and bolus obstruction.

Cervical webs

These usually occur anteriorly in the postcricoid region. They are more common in females, sometimes associated with iron deficiency and may complicate bullous conditions (Chapter 13) and graft versus host disease (Chapter 16).

The webs can usually be diagnosed by careful contrast radiology. However, in practice they are often first detected endoscopically. Often they can be ruptured quite simply just by passing the endoscope, but occasionally bougies or balloon rupture is necessary.

Mid-oesophageal webs

These are uncommon. Some are idiopathic, but more often they complicate bullous conditions and graft versus host disease. Diagnosis and treatment is as for cervical webs.

RINGS

By far the commonest type of lesion is the lower oesophageal (Schatzki) ring. This usually occurs at the squamocolumnar junction. Most cases are probably asymptomatic but they may cause intermittent short-lived solid food dysphagia, especially if food ingestion has been hurried. A ring less than 13 mm in diameter is said to always result in dysphagia, but this does not occur if the diameter is more than 20 mm [9].

Gastro-oesophageal reflux can often be demonstrated, but is rarely symptomatic [10].

The diagnosis is best made radiologically, using a solid contrast meal in the upright posture and achieving maximal distension of the oesophagus. Endoscopically Schatzki rings are easily missed unless the oesophagus is distended with air.

These lesions often require no treatment other than the patient adjusting his/her eating habits accordingly. However, they may be ruptured by bougie or balloon, although they often recur [11].

DIVERTICULA

Pharyngeal pouch (Zenker's diverticulum)

A pharyngeal pouch is the commonest type of oesophageal diverticulum. They occur chiefly in the midline between the inferior pharyngeal constrictor and cricopharyngeus muscles, but may also occur at other sites of potential weakness in the muscle layer. They are probably due to pulsion forces secondary to a restrictive myopathy of the cricopharyngeus muscle that reduces upper oesophageal sphincter compliance and opening [12,13] (p. 101).

Characteristically a pharyngeal pouch presents after the age of 50 with dysphagia, regurgitation, cough, spluttering, aspiration, choking, a bulge in the neck and bad breath. The regurgitated food may be that ingested many hours before. Eventually weight loss may occur.

Unusual complications include carcinoma [14], ulceration [15], fistula [16] and haemorrhage [17].

The diagnosis is made radiologically, the findings being quite characteristic (Figure 14.2).

Treatment is now usually carried out by ENT surgeons using an endoscopic stapling device to create a common cavity between the pouch and oesophagus [18].

Mid-oesophageal diverticulum

Mid-oesophageal diverticula are rarely symptomatic, but if very large may result in regurgitation. They may occur by traction from tuberculous mediastinal nodes, or occur in association with spastic motility disorders of the oesophagus [19].

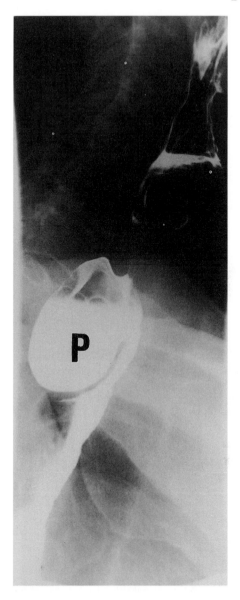

Figure 14.2 Lateral view of barium swallow showing a large pharyngeal pouch (P).

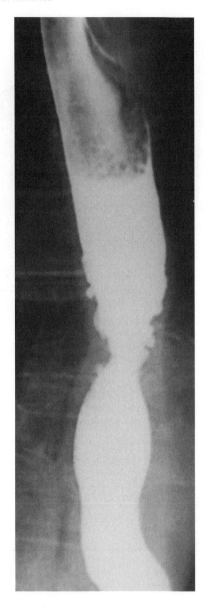

Figure 14.3 Barium swallow illustrating pseudodiverticulosis. Note the numerous tiny outpouchings in the mid-oesophagus. This patient also had endoscopic oesophagitis.

Epiphrenic diverticulum

These are usually associated with oesophageal motility disorders. They are often multiple and rarely *per se* cause symptoms [19]. Rarely they may perforate, fistulate or bleed. They rarely need treatment.

Intramural pseudodiverticulosis

This is a rare condition usually occurring in the sixth or seventh decades. It is characterized by generalized or segmental tiny flask-shaped out-pouchings of the oesophageal epithelium (Figure 14.3). The lesions are due to dilated ducts of the submucosal glands [20]. The cause is unknown, but the condition is often associated with reflux oesophagitis, *Candida*, diabetes or neoplasm [21].

The most common presenting symptom is dysphagia. The diagnosis is made radiologically. There may be associated long strictures. Rarely the openings of the diverticula can be seen endoscopically [22].

Any associated condition needs to be treated. Strictures may require dilatation.

REFERENCES

1. Ott DJ. Gastroesophageal reflux: what is the role of barium studies? *AJR* 1994; **162**: 627–629.
2. Windsor CWO, Collis JL. Anaemia and hiatus hernia: experience in 450 patients. *Thorax* 1967; **22**: 73–78.
3. Cameron AJ, Higgins JA. Linear gastric erosion. *Gastroenterology* 1986; **91**: 338–342.
4. Boyd EJS, Penston JG, Russell RI, Wormsley KG *et al*. Hiatal hernia ulcers: clinical features and follow-up. *Postgrad Med J* 1991; **67**: 900–903.
5. Moskovitz M, Fadden R, Min T *et al*. Large hiatal hernias, anemia, and linear gastric erosion: studies of etiology and medical therapy. *Am J Gastroenterol* 1992; **87**: 622–626.
6. Hill LD. Incarcerated paraesophageal hernia – a surgical emergency. *Am J Surg* 1973; **126**: 286–291.
7. Haas O, Rat P, Christoph M *et al*. Surgical results of intrathoracic gastric volvulus complicating hiatal hernia. *Br J Surg* 1990; **77**: 1379–1381.
8. Wo JM, Branum GD, Hunter JG *et al*. Clinical features of type III (mixed) paraesophageal hernia. *Am J Gastroenterol* 1996; **91**: 914–916.

9. Schatzki R. The lower esophageal ring: long-term follow-up of symptomatic and asymptomatic rings. *AJR* 1963; **90**: 805–810.

10. Marshall JB, Kretschmar JM, Kiaz-Arias AA. Gastroesophageal reflux as a pathogenic factor in the development of symptomatic lower esophageal rings. *Arch Intern Med* 1990; **150**: 1669–1672.

11. Eckardt VF, Kanzler G, Willems D. Single dilation of symptomatic Schatzki rings. A prospective evaluation of its effectiveness. *Dig Dis Sci* 1992; **37**: 577–582.

12. Cook IJ, Blumbergs P, Cash K *et al.* Structural abnormalities of the cricopharyngeus muscle in patients with pharyngeal (Zenker's) diverticulum. *J Gastroenterol Hepatol* 1992; **7**: 556–562.

13. Cook IJ, Gabb M, Panagopoulos V *et al.* Pharyngeal (Zenker's) diverticulum is a disorder of upper esophageal sphincter opening. *Gastroenterology* 1992; **103**: 1229–1235.

14. Bowdler DA, Stell PM. Carcinoma arising in posterior pharyngeal pulsion diverticulum (Zenker's diverticulum). *Br J Surg* 1987; **74**: 561–563.

15. Shirazi KK, Daffner RH, Gaede JT. Ulcer occurring in Zenker's diverticulum. *Gastrointest Radiol* 1977; **2**: 117–118.

16. Stanford W, Barloon TJ, Lu CC. Esophagotracheal fistula from a pharyngoesophageal diverticulum. *Chest* 1983; **84**: 229–231.

17. Hendren WG, Anderson T, Miller JI. Massive bleeding in a Zenker's diverticulum. *South Med J* 1990; **83**: 362.

18. Mahieu HF, de Bree R, Dagli SA, Snel AM. The pharyngoesophageal segment: endoscopic treatment of Zenker's diverticulum. *Dis Esoph* 1996; **9**: 12–21.

19. Rivkin L, Bremner CG, Bremner CH. Pathophysiology of mid-oesophageal and epiphrenic diverticula of the oesophagus. *S Afr Med J* 1984; **66**: 127–129.

20. Lupovitch A, Tippins R. Esophageal intramural pseudodiverticulosis: a disease of adnexal glands. *Radiology* 1974; **113**: 271–272.

21. Cho SR, Sanders MM, Turner MA *et al.* Esophageal intramural pseudodiverticulosis. *Gastrointest Radiol* 1981; **6**: 9–16.

22. Van der Putten ABMM, Loffeld RJLF. Esophageal intramural pseudo-diverticulosis. *Dis Esoph* 1997; **10**: 61–63.

15

Traumatic conditions

Perforation of the oesophagus as a result of instrumentation, ulcers or other specific pathological processes is discussed elsewhere (Chapters 5, 8, 12 and 16).

Mallory–Weiss tears, spontaneous rupture, intramural rupture and intramural haematoma are four traumatic conditions of the oesophagus that have several features in common. Other conditions to be discussed in this chapter include mucosal prolapse, foreign bodies and oesophageal casts.

MALLORY–WEISS TEAR

A Mallory–Weiss tear is relatively common, accounting for more than 10% of the causes of acute haematemesis and/or melaena [1,2]. The lesion is a small linear tear above, at or below the oesophagogastric junction. It occurs more commonly in the presence of a hiatus hernia.

Characteristically it is associated with vomiting and almost certainly results from the forces at the oesophagogastric junction during the vomiting process [2]. Although haematemesis may follow non-bloody emesis it is more common for blood to be present with the first vomit [2]. There may be associated low retrosternal/upper epigastric pain. Usually the patients are male and have often been consuming alcohol heavily. The amount of haemorrhage is usually relatively minor, but it may be massive and require interventional therapy such as injection, coagulation or suturing.

Diagnosis is made easily by endoscopy, which reveals the characteristic linear tear.

SPONTANEOUS RUPTURE OF THE OESOPHAGUS (BOERHAAVE'S SYNDROME)

Spontaneous rupture of the oesophagus is a serious medical/surgical emergency in which prompt diagnosis is essential for a reasonable chance of survival. Unfortunately, diagnosis is often delayed.

The lesion consists of a linear tear through the full thickness of the lateral (usually left) wall of the oesophagus just above the diaphragm. It usually occurs after forceful and sudden vomiting, but occasionally after coughing or even straining at stool [3]. There is often a history of heavy drinking and many patients have an associated peptic ulcer [4] (Figure 15.1).

In addition to vomiting the patient usually presents with severe lower chest/epigastric/left upper abdominal pain which may radiate through to the back. There may also be dyspnoea and shock.

On examination there may be little to find initially other than the fact the patient is in severe pain, but soon the signs of left pleural effusion emerge. Emphysema in the neck is a later sign.

The initial differential diagnosis includes myocardial infarction, dissecting aneurysm, pneumonia, perforated peptic ulcer and acute pancreatitis.

A straight X-ray early after presentation may reveal air in the mediastinum, or under the left parietal pleura and above the left diaphragm. Later there will be a hydropneumothorax. Analysis of the pleural fluid for pH and amylase may be helpful. Occasionally a careful radiological contrast swallow may be needed to confirm the diagnosis. Unless the rupture is very small surgical intervention is almost invariably necessary. The prognosis is very much dependent upon timing of surgery. If this is carried out within 12 hours mortality may be below 25% but it may be above 75% if surgery is delayed for more than 48 hours [4].

SPONTANEOUS INTRAMURAL RUPTURE

This condition is characterized by a longitudinal tear extending from the mucosa, but not sufficient to cause perforation. The lesions may be extensive in length, but usually occur away from the gastro-oesophageal junction. There is often extensive bruising and haematoma formation.

In contrast to spontaneous rupture of the oesophagus there is usually no history of forceful vomiting [5]. The cause is usually obscure. The presenting symptoms are severe retrosternal pain, odynophagia and dysphagia. These are followed by haematemesis, which may be delayed for some hours [5].

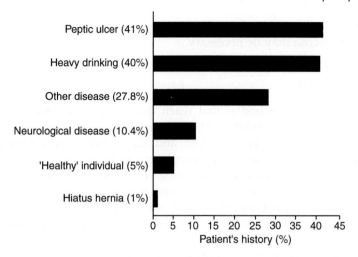

Figure 15.1 Conditions associated with spontaneous rupture of the oesophagus. This analysis is based on 349 patients from multiple published series. (Source: redrawn from reference 4, with permission of the publisher.)

The diagnosis is usually obvious at endoscopy, the tear and haematoma being easily recognizable.

With conservative management the prognosis is good [5].

INTRAMURAL HAEMATOMA

Intramural haematoma is a condition with striking similarities to intramural rupture except that there is no extensive mucosal laceration. Although some cases follow forceful vomiting or are associated with a bleeding diathesis many are idiopathic [6].

The presentation is very similar to that of intramural rupture, with chest pain, dysphagia and sometimes overt bleeding. Endoscopically the haematoma is easily recognized and often very extensive. There may be points of bleeding breaking through the mucosa.

The prognosis is excellent provided that any underlying bleeding disorder is appropriately corrected.

MUCOSAL PROLAPSE

Endoscopists are familiar with prolapse of the gastric mucosa into the oesophagus while patients are retching. Usually this is of no clinical significance, but prolapsed mucosa may become engorged, ulcerated and even incarcerated [7–9]. With these complications the patients may complain of pain or experience haematemesis. Surgical resection of the prolapsed mucosa may be necessary.

FOREIGN BODY

Most ingested foreign bodies that reach the stomach pass through the alimentary tract uneventfully [10]. The problem occurs particularly in children, the mentally handicapped and the elderly. The commonest 'foreign bodies' to obstruct in the oesophagus include meat (especially in association with oesophageal diseases), coins, button batteries and pills/tablets (Chapter 16). The commonest sites of obstruction are at the level of the cricopharyngeus, above the aortic arch, in the lower oesophagus or above sites of organic obstruction. Characteristically the patient complains of pain, dysphagia and odynophagia. There may be excessive salivation, regurgitation and vomiting.

Depending on the nature of the object it may be visible on straight X-ray (posteroanterior and lateral views). Contrast radiology can also be helpful, but must be undertaken cautiously for fear of aspiration. In practice the diagnosis is usually suspected clinically and confirmed endoscopically.

The treatment of choice is endoscopic removal [11], with use of an overtube for sharp objects [12]. The procedure may sometimes need to be carried out under general anaesthetic in order to protect the airway.

Complications arising from foreign bodies in the oesophagus include haemorrhage, perforation, aspiration, the effects of leakage from button batteries [13] and the caustic effects of pills/tablets (Chapter 16).

OESOPHAGEAL CASTS

This is a rare condition characterized by vomiting a tubular oesophageal cast consisting of squamous mucosa, the distal end sometimes remaining attached. It occurs particularly after ingestion of very hot drinks [14].

REFERENCES

1. Knauer CM. Mallory–Weiss syndrome. *Gastroenterology* 1976; **71**: 5–8.
2. Graham DY, Schwartz JT. The spectrum of Mallory–Weiss tear. *Medicine* 1977; **57**: 307–318.
3. Henderson JAM, Peloquin AJM. Boerhaave's revisited: spontaneous esophageal perforation as a masquerader. *Am J Med* 1986; **86**: 559–567.
4. Brauer RB, Liebermann-Meffert D, Stein HJ *et al.* Boerhaave's

syndrome: analysis of the literature and report of 18 new cases. *Dis Esoph* 1997; **10**: 64–68.

5. Steadman C, Kerlin P, Crimmins F *et al.* Spontaneous intramural rupture of the oesophagus. *Gut* 1990; **31**: 845–849.
6. Fraser A, Masson J, Phull PS *et al.* Extensive intramural haematoma of the oesophagus. *Gastroenterology* 1997;112: A119.
7. Palmer ED. Mucosal prolapse at the esophagogastric junction. *Am J Gastroenterol* 1955; **23**: 530–537.
8. DeLorimier AA, Warren JP. Prolapse of the mucosa at the esophagogastric junction. *AJR* 1960; **84**: 1061–1069.
9. Blum SD, Weiss A, Weiselberg HM *et al.* Retrograde prolapse of gastric mucosa into the oesophagus. *Gastroenterology* 1961; **41**: 408–411.
10. Selivanov V, Sheldon GF, Cello JP *et al.* Management of foreign body ingestion. *Ann Surg* 1984; **199**: 187–191.
11. Berggreen PJ, Harrison E, Sanowski RA *et al.* Techniques and complications of esophageal foreign body extraction in children and adults. *Gastrointest Endosc* 1993; **39**: 626–630.
12. Spurling TJ, Zaloga GP, Richter JE. Fibre-endoscopic removal of a gastric foreign body with an overtube technique. *Gastrointest Endosc* 1983; **29**: 226–227.
13. Studley JGN, Linehan IP, Ogilvie AL, Dowling BL. Swallowed button batteries: is there a consensus on management? *Gut* 1990; **31**: 867–870.
14. Stevens AE, Dove JAW. Oesophageal cast, oesophagitis dissecans superficialis. *Lancet* 1960; **ii**: 1279–1280.

16

Miscellaneous inflammatory conditions

NON-STEROIDAL ANTI-INFLAMMATORY DRUGS (NSAIDs)

The harmful effect of NSAIDs on the gastroduodenal mucosa, including superficial and deep ulceration, are well known. The mechanism is at least partly due to prostaglandin synthatase inhibition, prostaglandins being important in maintaining integrity of the mucosa against acid–peptic damage.

In the oesophagus ingestion of NSAIDs has also been associated with ulceration and stricture formation (Chapter 5) [1,2]. The mechanism for damage is probably not like that in the gastroduodenal mucosa as endogenous levels of oesophageal mucosal prostaglandins are normally extremely low or undetectable [3]. Many patients [1], but by no means all [2], have underlying abnormalities such as gastro-oesophageal reflux or a Schatzki ring, which may result in the lodging of the pill/tablet in the lower oesophagus to cause damage by a local corrosive action.

In the setting of gastro-oesophageal reflux, particularly with oesophagitis, high levels of prostaglandin E_2 (PGE_2) have been found in the oesophageal mucosa [3]. PGE_2 itself appears to have no direct effect on the oesophageal mucosa, either protective or damaging. However, it can reduce lower oesophageal sphincter pressure and might therefore enhance reflux, which would aggravate oesophageal damage and lead to a 'vicious cycle' [4]. Morgan [4] has suggested that NSAIDs could, paradoxically, be therapeutically useful in this situation as they might prevent the PGE_2-induced relaxation of the sphincter. A proton-pump inhibitor would have to be given simultaneously to heal the underlying oesophagitis. This interesting concept awaits evaluation.

PILLS/TABLET DAMAGE

Apart from NSAIDs many other medications may cause oesophageal damage, in particular tetracyclines, other antibiotics, emepronium bromide, potassium chloride, ferrous sulphate, beta-blockers, antimalarials and biphosphonates [5].

The problem occurs particularly in the elderly or when insufficient fluid is taken to carry the medication into the stomach. The usual sites of obstruction include just above the aortic arch or lower oesophageal sphincter and above any organic obstruction. Damage is usually due to a direct toxic effect of the medication.

Symptoms include pain, odynophagia, dysphagia, bleeding and perforation. The patient may have been aware of the pill/tablet sticking in the oesophagus.

Endoscopically the changes include focal erythema, superficial or deep ulcers and stricture.

Treatment should consist of withdrawing the medication, at least until the lesions have healed. Strictures may require dilatation (Chapter 5). The patient must be educated about the importance of taking adequate fluid with pills/tablets.

CAUSTIC DAMAGE

Caustic damage to the oesophagus usually occurs accidentally in children or as a suicide attempt in adults. Both alkalis and acids may cause oesophageal corrosion. The mouth and stomach will also often be involved. Damage may be severe with total sloughing of the mucosa and even full-thickness necrosis. With recovery there may be extensive stricture formation, which may be complicated by carcinoma [6].

Acutely the patient presents with severe pain, odynophagia, bleeding, salivation and fever. There may be respiratory distress from laryngeal oedema. If the oesophagus has perforated the patient will be desperately ill.

Although endoscopy is potentially dangerous most authors agree this should be carried out at an early stage to assess the extent of damage. The endoscopic appearances include erythema, superficial or deep ulceration, exudate, perforation and necrotic mucosa [7].

The immediate treatment, depending on the severity of the oesophageal damage, includes pain relief, establishing an adequate airway and intravenous fluids. Emetics should be avoided because of the risk of a second oesophageal exposure to the damaging material. Urgent surgical intervention will be necessary for perforation or oesophageal necrosis. Corticosteroids are of no value [8]. If the patient recovers, endoscopic surveillance should be carried out after 2–3 weeks to assess and treat strictures. Repeated stricture dilatations may be necessary.

EOSINOPHILIC OESOPHAGITIS

A distinct condition of eosinophilic oesophagitis has been described [9]. Although the oesophageal mucosa looks entirely normal endoscopically, biopsies show a dense eosinophil infiltration within the squamous epithelium of the oesophagus (> 50 eosinophils/high power field), together with papillary and basal zone hyperplasia.

The condition particularly affects young males. The clinical presentation is episodic dysphagia, but there is no radiologically demonstrable obstruction. Oesophageal manometry often shows minor non-specific abnormalities. There is no associated gastro-oesophageal reflux as assessed by oesophageal pH monitoring. Some patients have a history of allergic conditions, but peripheral blood eosinophilia is unusual. The dysphagia responds to oesophageal dilatations, which may have to be repeated, or corticosteroids.

The relationship to eosinophilic gastroenteritis is unclear. Undoubtedly some patients present with dominant oesophageal symptoms, but oesophageal involvement can also occur in eosinophilic gastroenteritis with lower alimentary involvement [10].

GRAFT VERSUS HOST DISEASE

Following bone marrow transplantation oesophageal damage can occur as part of multisystem chronic graft versus host disease – 13% of 105 patients in one series [11].

The characteristic presenting symptoms are odynophagia/dysphagia. Endoscopy reveals desquamation, which may heal with webs, rings or strictures [11].

RADIATION OESOPHAGITIS

Odynophagia and/or dysphagia are almost invariable during mediastinal radiotherapy [12]. Structural damage such as mucosal injury, stricture and fistula is much less common and dose-dependent [13]. The mechanism for oesophageal symptoms in those without injury is uncertain, but does not appear to be altered motility [12]. Treatment is symptomatic.

GLYCOGENIC ACANTHOSIS/LEUCOPLAKIA

Small (< 4 mm), whitish, slightly raised discrete plaques, often multiple in number, are found in the oesophagus in 2% of endoscopic examinations. PAS staining often reveals an increased glycogen content. They are therefore often referred to as glycogenic acanthosis [14]. They are of no clinical significance other than that they must be differentiated from candidal plaques.

Larger lesions, usually termed leucoplakia, may also be found [15].

NECROTIZING OESOPHAGITIS

This is a rare condition and not due to caustic damage. It occurs particularly in critical ill patients and may be due to ischaemia. Endoscopically the mucosa is diffusely blackened and there may be exudate, ulcers and haemorrhage [16]. The prognosis is usually that of the underlying disorder. There is no specific treatment.

CROHN'S DISEASE

Involvement of the oesophagus in Crohn's disease is rare, but when present it affects particularly the mid and lower zones. The appearances are of Crohn's disease elsewhere, i.e. ulceration, cobblestoning and stricturing [17].

REFERENCES

1. Heller SR, Fellowes IW, Ogilvie AL, Atkinson M. Non-steroidal anti-inflammatory drugs and benign oesophageal stricture. *Br Med J* 1982; **285**: 167–168.
2. El-Serag HB, Sonnenberg A. Association of esophagitis and esophageal strictures with diseases treated with non-steroidal anti-inflammatory drugs. *Am J Gastroenterol* 1997; **92**: 52 -56.
3. Long JD, Orlando RC. Eicosanoids and the esophagus. *Dig Dis* 1997; **15**: 145–154.
4. Morgan GP. Therapeutic potential of NSAIDs and omeprazole in the oesophagus. *Scand J Gastroenterol* 1997; **32**: 95.
5. Kikendall JW, Johnson LF. Pill-induced esophageal injury. In: Castell DO, ed. *The Esophagus.* 2nd ed. Boston, MA: Little, Brown, 1995: pp 619–633.
6. Appelquist P, Salmo N. Lye corrosive strictures of the esophagus – a review of 63 cases. *Cancer* 1980; **45**: 2655–2658.
7. Di Costanzo J, Noirclerc M, Jouclard J *et al.* New therapeutic approach to corrosive burns of the upper gastrointestinal tract. *Gut* 1980; **21**: 370–375.
8. Anderson KD, Rouse TM, Randolph JG. A controlled trial of corticosteroids in children with corrosive injury of the esophagus. *N Engl J Med* 1990; **323**: 637–640.
9. Attwood SEA, Smyrk TC, De Meester TR, Jones JB. Esophageal

eosinophilia with dysphagia. A distinct clinical pathologic syndrome. *Dig Dis Sci* 1993; **38**: 109–116.

10. Dobbins JW, Sheahan DG, Behar J. Eosinophilic gastroenteritis with esophageal involvement. *Gastroenterology* 1977; **72**: 1312–1316.
11. McDonald GB, Sullivan KM, Plumley TF. Radiographic features of esophageal involvement in chronic graft-versus-host disease. *AJR* 1984; **142**: 501–506.
12. Yeoh E, Holloway RH, Russo A *et al*. Effects of mediastinal irradiation on oesophageal function. *Gut* 1996; **38**: 166–170.
13. Lepke RA, Libshitz HI. Radiation-induced injury of the esophagus. *Radiology* 1983; **148**: 375–378.
14. Blackstone MO. The esophagus – variations from the normal appearance. In: *Endoscopic Interpretation: I. The Esophagus*, New York: Raven Press, 1984: pp 14–18.
15. Lam TS, Lack E, Benjamin SB. Compact parakeratosis of esophageal mucosa: a non-specific lesion mimicking 'leukoplakia'. *Gastrointest Endosc* 1990; **36**: 397–399.
16. Goldenberg SP, Wain SL, Marignaini P. Acute necrotising esophagitis. *Gastroenterology* 1990; **98**: 493–496.
17. Huchzermeyer H, Paul F, Seifert E *et al*. Endoscopic results in five patients with Crohn's disease of the esophagus. *Endoscopy* 1976; **8**: 75–81.

17

Rumination

CLINICAL FEATURES

Rumination is characterized by regurgitation of recently ingested food into the mouth, remastication and reswallowing. The cycle is often repeated until the regurgitated food becomes acidic, usually about 30 minutes after commencing the meal. The process is not unpleasant for the patient and may even be pleasurable [1]. Some patients complain of weight loss, nausea, abdominal discomfort and heartburn, but these are unusual [2,3].

There may be underlying mental retardation or psychiatric disorders, but the condition may also affect apparently normal adults [4]. In the latter group there is often a history of a psychologically or physically stressful episode [4].

The pathophysiology is unclear. Oesophageal motility, gastric emptying and electrogastrography have all been reported as normal [4].

The condition may be mistaken particularly for gastro-oesophageal reflux, achalasia, oesophageal stricture, gastric outlet obstruction and gastroparesis.

Although the condition may persist for many years the ultimate prognosis is good. A variety of psychotherapeutic manoeuvres have been used, including relaxation therapy and biofeedback [4].

REFERENCES

1. Richter JE. Functional esophageal disorders. In: Drossman DA, ed. *The Functional Gastrointestinal Disorders*. Boston, MA: Little, Brown, 1994: pp 25–70.
2. O'Brien MD, Bruce BK, Camilleri M. The rumination syndrome: clinical features rather than manometric diagnosis. *Gastroenterology* 1995; **108**: 1024–1029.
3. Shay SS, Johnson LF, Wong RKH *et al*. Rumination, heartburn and daytime gastroesophageal reflux. *J Clin Gastroenterol* 1986; **8**: 115–126.

4. Soykan I, Chen J, Kendall BJ, McCallum RW. The rumination syndrome. Clinical and manometric profile, therapy, and long-term outcome. *Dig Dis Sci* 1997; **42**: 1866–1872.

18

Dysphagia

Although the specific conditions causing dysphagia have been described in relevant previous chapters, it is a common and often serious symptom requiring a disciplined approach to both history-taking and investigation for accurate diagnosis. The purpose of this chapter is to outline the principles involved and list the differential diagnoses.

A careful history is essential. Dysphagia means difficulty with swallowing and should not be confused with odynophagia (painful swallowing), although both symptoms often occur simultaneously. True dysphagia can be usefully classified into oropharyngeal (affecting the mouth, pharynx and upper oesophageal sphincter) and oesophageal (affecting the body of the oesophagus and lower oesophageal sphincter/cardia of the stomach). Various painful conditions of the mouth are sometimes listed as causes of dysphagia, but are really causes of odynophagia. These include infections (e.g. *Candida*, herpes), inflammatory conditions (Crohn's, Behçet's), bullous disorders, painful conditions of the teeth and gums, trauma and tumours.

Oropharyngeal dysphagia (Table 18.1) is usually a problem of initiating swallowing and is sometimes referred to as 'transfer dysphagia'. The patient complains of food sticking in the throat and there may be associated nasal regurgitation, coughing, spluttering and choking on swallowing. There will often be symptoms and signs of the underlying disease process (Table 18.1). It must not be confused with globus sensation, a feeling of a lump in the throat, which is usually constant and may be associated with a sensation of a need to swallow.

With oesophageal dysphagia (Table 18.2) there is usually a delay of a few seconds after swallowing before the dysphagia is experienced. Even with true low oesophageal causes about one-third of patients localize the sensation of obstruction to the neck [1].

Dysphagia associated with oesophageal motility disorders is often

Table 18.1   Causes of oropharyngeal dysphagia

- Mechanical (intrinsic) – pharyngeal pouch (Zenker's diverticulum), tumour, web, radiation fibrosis
- Mechanical (extrinsic) – thyroid, abscess, other extrinsic masses, cervical spondylosis
- Muscular–impaired cricopharyngeal muscle opening, myasthenia gravis, myositis, muscular dystrophy, thyroid disease
- Neurological – stroke, Parkinson's, motor neuron disease, cerebral palsy, brain tumour, multiple sclerosis, poliomyelitis, peripheral and autonomic neuropathies
- Infective – *Candida*, herpes simplex, cytomegalovirus, tuberculosis, tonsillitis
- Xerostomia – any cause of dry mouth

Table 18.2   Causes of oesophageal dysphagia

- Mechanical (intrinsic) – tumour, ring, web, stricture, foreign body
- Mechanical (extrinsic) – vascular (aorta, aberrant vessels, enlarged left atrium), mediastinal nodes/masses
- Primary motility disorders – achalasia, diffuse oesophageal spasm, nutcracker oesophagus, hypertensive lower oesophageal sphincter, non-specific oesophageal motility disorder, ?failed secondary peristalsis, ?reduced traction force during primary peristalsis
- Secondary motility disorders – scleroderma, other connective tissue diseases, Chagas' disease
- Inflammatory – gastro-oesophageal reflux, drug-induced oesophagitis, eosinophilic oesophagitis
- Infective – *Candida*, herpes simplex, cytomegalovirus, tuberculosis, other bacterial infections, HIV ulcer

characterized by difficulty in swallowing both liquids and solids, whereas with mechanical obstruction solids are at least initially more troublesome. Intermittent dysphagia over a period of many months or years is characteristic of obstruction due to a web or ring. Rapidly progressive dysphagia often indicates underlying malignancy.

INVESTIGATIONS

A straight chest X-ray is sometimes helpful. This may reveal a variety of relevant problems, including tumours, goitre, aortic aneurysm, large left atrium, abnormalities typical of achalasia and evidence of respiratory spill-over.

After indirect pharyngoscopy, suspected oropharyngeal dysphagia should be investigated with a rapid-sequence videorecorded barium swallow with both anteroposterior and lateral projections. Playback in slow motion will often reveal the underlying mechanism. Co-operation and communication between clinician and radiologist is essential. Upper oesophageal manometry is not routinely applicable [2], but may become so with improved recording equipment [3].

A barium swallow is usually the first line of investigation for suspected oesophageal dysphagia. Again, co-operation with radiologists is essential. Different techniques may be required for different presentations. In addition to a liquid suspension it may be necessary to administer barium with a solid (bread or marshmallow) to reveal subtle obstructive lesions. A Schatzki ring may only be revealed by a fully distended oesophagus in the upright posture, sometimes together with a Valsalva manoeuvre. It may be necessary to carry out the swallow in the supine posture to reveal motility disorders. If the barium swallow is negative, endoscopy is usually the next investigation of choice as mucosal abnormalities may not be revealed by contrast radiology. If an obstructive lesion has been identified by radiology, endoscopy will usually be required for biopsy. Some investigators prefer to perform endoscopy for oesophageal dysphagia without prior radiology, but this should not be the initial investigation for suspected oropharyngeal dysphagia for fear of intubating and rupturing a pharyngeal pouch or perforating the pharynx above a high obstruction. Oesophageal manometry is indicated if both contrast radiology and endoscopy are negative or to clarify the nature of a suspected motility disorder on the basis of previous investigations. Oesophageal scintigraphy is sometimes a useful complementary investigation (Chapter 19).

REFERENCES

1. Edwards DAW, Lobello R. Site of referral of the sense of obstruction to swallowing. *Gut* 1982; **23**: A435.
2. Ergun GA, Kahrilas PJ. Clinical applications of esophageal manometry and pH monitoring. *Am J Gastroenterol* 1996; **91**: 1077–1089.
3. Castell JA, Castell DO. Upper esophageal sphincter and pharyngeal function and oropharyngeal (transfer) dysphagia. *Gastroenterol Clin North Am* 1996; **25**: 35–50.

19

Specialist oesophageal investigations

Stationary manometry and 24-hour ambulatory pH monitoring have had a major impact on the diagnosis and management of oesophageal disorders. Their availability is an essential part of the provision of a comprehensive oesophageal service. Commercially available packages of equipment and computer software are now very 'user-friendly' and are easily set up in a district general hospital [1]. Combined ambulatory manometry/pH packages are now available and are beginning to establish a defined role. A system for measuring duodenogastro-oesophageal reflux (Bilitec) is also available and has been of considerable research interest, but has not so far proved to be of value in routine clinical practice.

Based on the known prevalence of oesophageal disorders, the Oesophageal Section of the British Society of Gastroenterology has calculated that 260 manometry and/or pH studies per year will be required for a population of 200 000. A full-time technician can be expected to perform 500 studies per year and could therefore provide a service for a population of approximately 400 000 [2].

OESOPHAGEAL MANOMETRY

Equipment

For assessment of oesophageal body function two types of catheter are available: water-perfused manometric assemblies and solid state intra-luminal transducers. Each has recording sites along the length of the catheter, usually at 3–5 cm intervals. The water-perfused systems are cheaper and more robust but somewhat cumbersome. The intraluminal transducers are often found to be more convenient to use.

For measurement of basal lower oesophageal sphincter pressure the catheter can be passed into the stomach and the pressure recorded as the sensor is pulled back through the sphincter. However, wide variations are found with time in individual subjects [3]. Furthermore, the sensor site measures only pressure in its immediate vicinity and it may be impossible to maintain its position, particularly during a swallow when the sphincter may move proximally by 2 cm [4]. Dent [5] has devised a perfused 6 cm recording sleeve to circumvent these problems. This has been shown to be particularly useful in assessing lower oesophageal sphincter relaxation, which is often necessary for the diagnosis of achalasia.

The procedure

Detailed accounts of carrying out oesophageal manometry are given elsewhere [6,7]. Only brief details will be outlined here. Primary peristalsis and sphincter relaxation are usually assessed with at least 10 × 5 ml water swallows, given at least 15 seconds apart. Secondary peristalsis can be assessed by introducing 10 ml boluses of air or water into a balloon in the mid-oesophagus [8].

Usefulness of oesophageal manometry

Stationary oesophageal manometry is undoubtedly of value or even essential in the diagnosis of achalasia and other motility disorders, including systemic sclerosis. Many regard manometric determination of the location of the sphincter as essential before carrying out 24-hour ambulatory pH recordings. Its value in 'tailoring' an anti-reflux operation is controversial (Chapter 4). It has been disappointing in the assessment of chest pain of uncertain cause (Chapter 10).

Indications for stationary oesophageal manometry [7,8]

- Diagnosis of non-obstructive dysphagia and other suspected motility disorders.
- To locate the lower oesophageal sphincter before pH recording.
- In the assessment of patients with gastro-oesophageal reflux who are being considered for anti-reflux surgery, particularly to exclude achalasia and systemic sclerosis.
- Rarely, in the assessment of chest pain of uncertain cause.

pH RECORDING

Equipment

Two types of recording electrode are in common use: glass and antimony. The glass electrodes have a linear response to changes in pH and are drift-free, but are bulky, fragile and relatively expensive. Antimony electrodes are easier for the patient, but can only be sterilized with isopropyl alcohol. They are less sensitive than glass electrodes, have a non-linear response and may show more drift. Despite their limitations, antimony electrodes are more often used in clinical practice.

The procedure

The catheter is passed transnasally and positioned 5 cm above the upper margin of the lower oesophageal sphincter, which should have been determined manometrically. During the recording period the patient should be encouraged to live as normally as possible but to avoid acid foods/drinks and antacids, and to have discontinued acid-suppressing therapy for at least 3 days beforehand. Further practical details are given in several recent reviews [8–10].

Analysis and limitations

pH monitoring records episodes of gastro-oesophageal reflux, including the extent of the change in oesophageal pH and its duration. What constitutes an episode of reflux and when these become abnormal is necessarily somewhat arbitrary. Defining reflux as an episode when the pH falls to less than 4 has stood the test of time as being clinically relevant [11,12]. However, particularly after meals when the pH of gastric contents may rise to more than 4, some episodes of reflux will not be detected. The upper limit of normal for the total duration of oesophageal pH < 4 during a 24-hour period ranged from 5–7% in one multicentre study [13]. Some groups have suggested differentiating upright and supine reflux, but this is of doubtful value (p. 16).

Combined intra-oesophageal and intragastric pH monitoring has been found to be particularly useful in assessing patients with a poor response to acid-suppressing therapy [14].

Several groups have interpreted oesophageal pH values of more than 7 to indicate duodenogastro-oesophageal reflux and refer to this as 'alkaline reflux'. This may be an erroneous interpretation of the data, the alkaline pH often being due to swallowed saliva or secretion of bicarbonate by the oesophageal mucosa [15]. Duodenogastro-oesophageal reflux can be determined using the bilirubin-sensing oesophageal probe (p. 161). The reproducibility of ambulant oesophageal pH monitoring is about 80% in patients with endoscopic oesophagitis [16,17] but less than this in endoscopy-negative patients or those with atypical symptoms [17]. It is unfortunate that reproducibility is not so good in the latter groups, since it is in these patients that the procedure would be of most diagnostic value.

Ideally episodes of recorded reflux should correlate with the patient's symptoms. Unfortunately a one-to-one match rarely exists. Various analyses have therefore been proposed including the symptom index [18]. This is defined as the percentage of symptom episodes associated with a fall in pH. Cut-off points of 50% and 75% have been suggested as diagnostic of abnormal reflux [8]. Unfortunately this index fails to take into account the number of reflux or symptom episodes, which may profoundly affect the analysis. Weusten *et al.* [19] have proposed measurement of the symptom-associated probability, a simple analysis based on Fisher's exact test, which does not have the above disadvantages. Unfortunately this is not yet available in commercial software packages.

Prolonged ambulant oesophageal pH monitoring is often considered the gold standard for the diagnosis of gastro-oesophageal reflux. Although undoubtedly the most accurate test available, its limitations must not be forgotten. The procedure is sometimes unpleasant and the associated stress/discomfort is likely to affect the recording. There may be technical problems, particularly drift with antimony electrodes that have been used several times. Problems with the analysis have been highlighted above. Finally, it is now recognized that a group of patients may have a normal total 24-hour oesophageal acid exposure, but show a good correlation between episodes of recorded reflux and symptoms ('hypersensitive oesophagus') and some even have endoscopic oesophagitis (p. 2) [20,21].

Indications for pH recording [8,9]

- Endoscopy-negative reflux type symptoms following a failed therapeutic trial of a proton-pump inhibitor.
- For confirmation of reflux in an endoscopy-negative patient being considered for anti-reflux surgery.
- To objectively assess response to medical or surgical treatment if a patient fails to achieve symptom improvement.
- To assess chest pain of uncertain origin or other atypical symptoms.

COMBINED MANOMETRY/pH RECORDING

Combined manometry/pH recording is now commercially available. It has been found to be useful in the diagnosis of chest pain of uncertain cause, but does not substantially increase the diagnostic yield above pH monitoring alone, acid reflux being a more common cause of the pain than motility disturbances (Chapter 10).

The procedure has been found to have good reproducibility in healthy volunteers [22].

ACID PERFUSION TEST

Forty years ago Bernstein and Baker [23] described the acid perfusion test as a measure of reproducing the pain of acid reflux. Physiological saline or 0.1 N hydrochloric acid are perfused alternatively into the patient's oesophagus in a patient blinded fashion. The test is positive if acid produces the patient's symptoms. Although the test has now been largely replaced by continuous ambulatory oesophageal pH monitoring, a recent study found a sensitivity of 100% and specificity of 73% when compared with pH monitoring [24]. If pH monitoring is not available the test is thus a reasonable 'second best'.

OESOPHAGEAL SCINTIGRAPHY

Some hospitals without oesophageal manometry/pH recording facilities will have a nuclear medicine department able to carry out oesophageal transit scintigraphy. Furthermore, in some patients oesophageal manometry is not tolerated or the results may be equivocal. Oesophageal manometry and scintigraphy measure different aspects of oesophageal function, scintigraphy being able to asses bolus transport [25].

The patient swallows 10 ml of water containing [^{99}Tc]-sulphur colloid while supine. The procedure may be repeated at 30-second intervals. It is also sometimes desirable to carry out the procedure with isotope-labelled solid boluses, particularly for the diagnosis of achalasia [26]. The oesophagus is divided into three 'regions of interest' (proximal, mid and distal) for construction of activity–time curves. In the absence of organic oesophageal obstruction and gastro-oesophageal reflux, 90% of the bolus is normally cleared from the oesophagus within 5–15 seconds [25].

Oesophageal scintigraphy may show characteristic abnormalities in achalasia, diffuse oesophageal spasm and other motility disorders [25].

REFERENCES

1. Donald IP, Ford GA, Wilkinson SP. Is 24-hour ambulatory oesophageal pH monitoring useful in a district general hospital? *Lancet* 1987; **i**: 89–91.
2. Watson A, Atkinson M. Provision of facilities for manometry and pH monitoring in the investigation of patients with oesophageal disease. *Gut* 1991; **32**: 106–107.
3. Dent J, Dodds WJ, Sekiguchi T *et al.* Interdigestive phasic contractions of the human lower esophageal sphincter. *Gastroenterology* 1983; **84**: 453–460.
4. Edmundowicz SA, Clouse RE. Shortening of the esophagus in response to swallowing. *Am J Physiol* 1991; **260**: G512-G516.

5. Dent J. A new technique for continuous sphincter pressure measurement. *Gastroenterology* 1976; **71**: 263–271.
6. Castell DO, Castell JA, eds. *Esophageal Motility Testing*. 2nd ed. Norwalk, CT: Appleton & Lange, 1994.
7. Ergun GA, Kahrilas PJ. Clinical applications of esophageal manometry and pH monitoring. *Am J Gastroenterol* 1996; **91**: 1077–1089.
8. Dent J, Holloway RH. Esophageal motility and reflux testing. State-of-the-art and clinical role in the twenty-first century. *Gastroenterol Clin North Am* 1996; **25**: 51–73.
9. Kahrilas PJ, Quigley EMM. Clinical esophageal pH recording: a technical review for practical guideline development. *Gastroenterology* 1996; **110**: 1982–1996.
10. Evans DF, Buckton GK. Clinical Measurements in Gastroenterology, vol 1. *The Oesophagus*. Oxford: Blackwell, 1997.
11. de Caestecker JS, Blackwell JN, Pryde A *et al.* Daytime gastro-oesophageal reflux is important in oesophagitis. *Gut* 1987; **28**: 519–529.
12. Joelsson B, Johnsson F. Heartburn – the acid test. *Gut* 1989; **30**: 1523–1525.
13. Richter JE, Bradley LA, DeMeester TR *et al.* Normal 24-hour ambulatory esophageal pH values: influence of study centre, pH electrode, age, and gender. *Dig Dis Sci* 1992; **37**: 849–856.
14. Klinkeenberg-Knol EC, Meuwissen SGM. Combined gastric and oesophageal 24-hour pH monitoring and oesophageal manometry in patients with reflux disease, resistant to treatment with omeprazole. *Aliment Pharmacol Ther* 1990; **4**: 485–495.
15. Singh S, Bradley LA, Richter JE. Determinants of oesophageal 'alkaline' pH environment in controls and patients with gastro-oesophageal reflux disease. *Gut* 1993; **34**: 309–316.
16. Johnsson F, Joelsson B. Reproduceability of ambulatory oesophageal pH monitoring. *Gut* 1988; **29**: 886–889.
17. Wiener GJ, Morgan TM, Cooper JB *et al.* Ambulatory 24-hour esophageal pH monitoring: reproduceability and variability of pH parameters. *Dig Dis Sci* 1988; **33**: 1127–1133.
18. Wiener GJ, Richter JE, Copper JB *et al.* The symptom index: a clinically important parameter of ambulatory 24-hour esophageal pH monitoring. *Am J Gastroenterol* 1988; **83**: 358–361.
19. Weusten BLAM, Roelfs JMM, Akkermans LMA *et al.* The symptom-association probability: an improved method for symptom analysis of 24-hour esophageal pH data. *Gastroenterology* 1994; **107**: 1741–1745.
20. Shi G, Bruley des Varannes S, Scarpignato C *et al.* Reflux related symptoms in patients with normal oesophageal exposure to acid. *Gut* 1995; **37**: 457–464.

21. Trimble KC, Douglas S, Pryde A *et al.* Clinical characteristics and natural history of symptomatic but not excess gastroesophageal reflux. *Dig Dis Sci* 1995; **40**: 1098–1104.
22. Wang H, Beck IT, Paterson WG. Reproduceability and physiological characteristics of 24-hour ambulatory esophageal manometry/pH-metry. *Am J Gastroenterol* 1996; **91**: 492–497.
23. Bernstein LM, Baker LA. A clinical test for esophagitis. *Gastroenterology* 1958; **34**: 760–781.
24. Howard PJ, Maher L, Pryde A, Heading RC. Symptomatic gastro-oesophageal reflux, abnormal oesophageal acid exposure, and mucosal acid sensitivity are three separate, though related, aspects of gastro-oesophageal reflux disease. *Gut* 1991; **32**: 128–132.
25. Kyriacou E, Heading RC. Oesophageal scintigraphy. In: Scarpignato C, Galmiche J-P, eds. *Functional Investigation in Esophageal Disease.* Basle: S Karger, 1994: pp 130–150.
26. Holloway RH, Krosin G, Lange RC *et al.* Radionuclide esophageal emptying of a solid meal to quantitate results of therapy in achalasia. *Gastroenterology* 1983; **84**: 771–776.

Index

abbreviation: CLO – columnar-lined oesophagus